A PRACTICAL GUIDE FOR

YOUNG ADULTS

A PRACTICAL GUIDE FOR

YOUNG ADULTS

CONSCIOUSLY CREATE
THE LIFE YOU'LL LOVE

Diana Hutchison

Illustrations by Lara Korotenko

A catalogue record for this book is available from the National Library of Australia

NATIONAL LIBRARY OF AUSTRALIA

The author of this book does not dispense medical advice or prescribe the use of any technique as a form of treatment, either directly or indirectly. The intent of the author is only to offer information of a general nature to help you in your quest for emotional and spiritual wellbeing. In the event you use any of the information in this book for yourself, which is your constitutional right, the author/publisher assume no responsibility for your actions. This book is not intended to be a substitute for the medical advice of a licensed physician. The reader should consult with their doctor in any matters relating to his/her health.

The material in this publication is of the nature of general comment only, and does not represent professional advice. It is not intended to provide specific guidance for particular circumstances and it should not be relied on as the basis for any decision to take action or not take action on any matter which it covers. Readers should obtain professional advice where appropriate, before making any such decision. To the maximum extent permitted by law, the author disclaims all responsibility and liability to any person, arising directly or indirectly from any person taking or not taking action based on the information in this publication.

ACKNOWLEDGEMENT

This book was conceived and written on the land of the Kaurna People.

We acknowledge and respect their spiritual relationship with their land and country. We also acknowledge the Kaurna People as the custodians of the Adelaide Plains region and that their cultural and heritage beliefs are important through all time.

We acknowledge and pay our respects to the cultural authority of past, present and emerging leaders and acknowledge and listen to their voices and messages for greater cultural inclusion.

CONTENTS

FREE DOWNLOADS

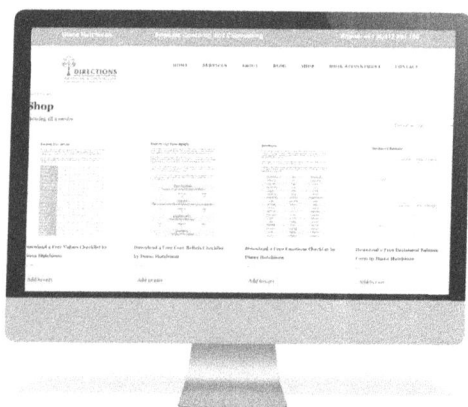

Grab your free downloads for self-assessment to accompany this book by visiting

www.dianahutchison.com/shop

PREFACE

This book is the second book in *The Practical Guide* series. While the books in this series are stand-alone books, you may find it helpful to have a copy of the first book, *A Practical Guide for Self Change,* to help you think about the steps that will begin to help you take action. Where *A Practical Guide for Self Change* looked at changing yourself and your life through creating your own self-change program, *A Practical Guide for Young Adults* explores many different areas of life and looks at how to get the best from each area of your life. If you manifest your potential, you will be creating an awesome you and giving yourself a pathway to living a purposeful life.

It is becoming more and more difficult to sort through the myriad of available information so that you can find the golden nuggets to help to build your life. This book provides a focus, so that you can take action to become your best, to fulfil your potential, and to create a wonderful life for yourself. *A Practical Guide for Young Adults* looks at the individual within a social setting. No one is isolated—we are all part of society and humanity.

Your beliefs and feelings determine where you put yourself within society and humanity.

I believe that it is difficult to isolate one part of us from all other parts, since we are integrated and complete beings. Although it is important to look at and explore all levels of being including the physical, emotional, mental and spiritual levels, this book will be specifically exploring areas of life and having that perspective. Further books in this series will go deeper into health and spiritual integration.

I thank the many people who contributed to this book. Whether through providing personal stories, feedback or both, you have made this book much more alive and all-encompassing. Thank you too to my editor, Hari Teah, who helped me to expand my mind and thoughts around what the book should talk about. A big thank you also to my mentor, Miriam Henke, who provided great feedback and has written the foreword.

Miriam is a health psychologist with special interests in mind-body medicine and photobiomodulation (PBM) therapy. She is also an executive coach and NLP Master Practitioner and Trainer. Miriam holds the title of Senior Clinical Lecturer at the University of Adelaide, and regularly contributes to innovation through research, supervision, and public speaking.

Thanks also go to my illustrator, Lara Korotenko, whose creativity and talent make the pages so much brighter.

Happy reading!

FOREWORD

_ BY MIRIAM HENKE

Adolescence and young adulthood are significant transitional periods in a person's life. A time of growing independence and learning about the responsibilities, joys, and pitfalls of adulthood. Milestones in previous generations, like, moving out of the family home, moving in with a partner, or getting married, are now being delayed until later in life. So, what's more important now to young people? According to the Australian Bureau of Statistics, young people are more interested in tertiary education (over half of young adults have non-school qualifications), being employed, travelling, and having rich social experiences.

This important time of life is complicated by the influence of cultural pressures, social media, the schooling system (that has a bias towards tertiary education and generally doesn't teach young people life skills), the allure of drugs and alcohol, and growing minds and bodies. A big part of this period of development is the importance placed on discovering one's own identity and sexuality, friendships, romantic relationships, and career paths. Young people are naturally quite self-absorbed and more likely to rebel against authority figures and parents in an effort to become their own person. This often leads to conflict with family and institutions (e.g., school, police), and can be a stressful time for those caring for the young person.

Parents, caregivers, and educators know all too well the realities of the world and what adulthood means. Their well-meaning efforts to rein in a young person's risky behaviours and *laissez-faire* attitudes inevitably butt heads with a young person's developing ideals, impulses, and values. It's a challenging time for everyone involved.

This book is a comprehensive set of guidelines for young people transitioning from childhood into adulthood; a time of great confusion, change, and pressure. What young people go through in their teenage years and early twenties is seriously intense. There's a lot to deal with day-to-day, let alone considering the future and what to do to prepare for the best future possible.

Being a teenager and young adult is easy for no one. Your body is changing, school is demanding and often a major drag, there's pressure on you from many sources (e.g., parents, teachers, friends, social media) to do well academically, in sports, in friendships, and for you to also contribute positively to your home and family life. Your teenage years are meant to be preparing you to become a functional adult in the "real world". However, many adults I know, including myself, felt that school simply didn't teach enough real-life skills.

Like all adults walking (or stumbling!) through life, we learn and figure things out as we go. Sometimes we get things right and sometimes we make mistakes. Life can be very hard. It can bring great suffering, pain, and torment. Knowing how to overcome obstacles, deal with your emotions and issues, bounce back after failure, heal a broken heart, and live on very little are all invaluable skills worth developing as early on as possible. Life can also give you the sweetest of thrills, pleasures, and priceless moments. Those delicious, fun, comforting, and beautiful things can bring both richness and reward, as well as addiction and escapism.

You'll find that people will give you lots and lots of advice at this time. Most you won't want, will disagree with, or completely ignore. There's a funny thing about the human mind that it will hear and take on the messages it needs, and it might need to be exposed to a particular message several times (and even over several years) before it gets taken in or acted on. We become awakened to ideas before we take them on, and if they appear to come from within us and align with our values, we're much more likely to act upon them.

I really believe Diana has written an extremely useful book to guide young people through the transition into adulthood with the information, wisdom, tools and tips needed to navigate a challenging yet incredibly rich time of life. This book is accessible, straightforward, judgement-free, and grounded in psychological research evidence. It's modern, relevant and will be a resource you can come back to time and again.

Without a doubt, a copy of this book will be gifted to each of my children on their 16th birthday. I want my kids to have something I didn't have when I was young, but something I wish I did have; the information not taught at school which you really need to truly be your best self and have an awesome life.

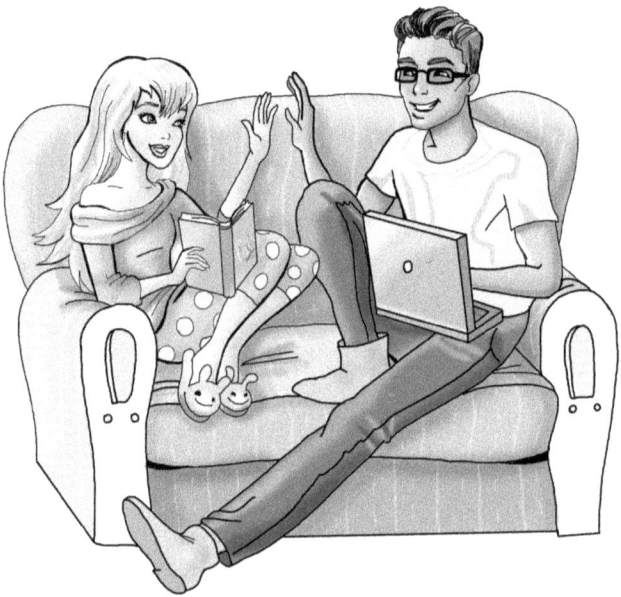

CHAPTER 1

HOW TO USE THIS BOOK

Welcome to *A Practical Guide for Young Adults* Each chapter explores a different area of life, and how to be the best in that area.

Before we begin, let me introduce myself. I have a background in psychology, and have now moved into counselling and life purpose coaching; helping people find their own unique self-healing pathway. I specialise in the areas of grief and loss, as well as health and wellbeing.

I have written this book because when I was a teenager and young adult, I felt like I could have really used the help and guidance a guide like this would have offered.

I believe gaining these insights during those years would have started me on the road to self-awareness and self-development much earlier in life. I hope that it helps you to explore the way you think and feel about your life, and how you want it to unfold.

Using these insights can really help you to make your life happen in the best way for you. It does take some effort, but if you are able to plan and organise things then it is likely to have positive effects.

Take charge of your life and don't allow your life to just happen to you – ensure *you* happen to *it*.

Taking action towards making small positive changes is the key.

The best way to use this book is to read it chapter by chapter.

You don't need to read the chapters in sequential order. You can read them in any order. Read a chapter, think about it, and if you have a friend or family member who is also reading it, then you could talk about it with them. It will be particularly helpful to do this if you are having some problems with the subjects discussed in that particular chapter.

If a family member or friend has recommended that you read this book, trust that they have your best interests at heart and give it a go.

Here is a short summary of how to approach each chapter, so that you get the most out of the book.

2. PHYSICAL HEALTH

After you have read through this chapter, go back and work out which areas you believe you can improve on in your life. It might be diet, it might be exercise, it might be both. You may not have thought about the long-term consequences of your behaviour, but find that you would like to do so now.

Maybe you'd like to stay healthy over the long term, and find that you are willing to think about putting different behaviours in place. It is your life and you can have a major impact on how it works out in the future. You now have the opportunity to change the way in which your life progresses.

Make a conscious decision to become authentic. Then you will be living the best life you could wish for, and later on you will be thankful that you made such a choice.

Read the chapter, check out the recommended websites and make a list of things you can do to effect change. To find help in goal setting and general aspects related to self-change, please refer to my previous book, *A Practical Guide for Self Change*.

You can download it from all book platforms, including Amazon. My amazon author page is: https://www.amazon.com/author/dianahutchison

3. HOME/FAMILY LIFE

After reading this chapter, think about your upbringing, your values and the beliefs you hold. Download the free *values* and *core beliefs* forms from my website www.dianahutchison.com/shop.

This will provide you with some information that you can act on, should you wish. Discuss your results with a family member or friend.

Think about where you fit into your family, school and wider community. Also consider your "in" group and "out" group. Your "in" group consists of a group of people whose characteristics mean that they get certain privileges. While society sets some of these, you can also set your own "in" group and "out" group, based on your ideas of inclusion and exclusion. Are you encompassing values of compassion for yourself and others?

4. RELATIONSHIPS

After reading through this chapter, consider the relationships you have right now and see them in the light of your feelings about them. Are they strong? Are they loving? Do you know them well?

Do you communicate well? Are you in a healthy relationship, or is it encroaching on your sense of self and not allowing you to breathe?

Get a sense of where you stand and where your relationships fit into your world.

5. SEX AND SEXUALITY

Reading this chapter will help you to form a clearer idea of your sexual needs and desires, so that you can form a healthy and positive sexual relationship with yourself and with others.

Communication is important so that you know where you stand, and so that you can ensure you and your partner are comfortable and happy with your choices.

Always ensure consent.

Whatever your sexual identity, orientation or preferences you are not alone.

Get support and ask for help when you need it.

6. INTERESTS AND HOBBIES

Make a note of the interests and hobbies that you really enjoy. This may give you an indication of the things that will stay with you through life or even point to something that might be a career. It would be helpful to explore your talents since these may well indicate the direction your career could go.

Not everybody knows their passions when they are young, but if you do, then factor these in to your life plans.

7. FINANCES

Reading this chapter will give you a base from which to start good money habits. Ensure you budget and work out your financial position. Then you'll have the ability to assess whether you can save some money for things you might want, rather than only ever having enough for the things you need. The important thing is to shop around for the best deal you can get.

Be realistic about what you can afford and take steps to ensure you are not spending more money than you have coming in. The exception to this is if you are on Social Security payments. There are ways of saving money that you can engage in. Investigate the suggestions outlined for you.

8. WORK/CAREER

When you read this chapter, think about what you came up with in Chapter 6.

Are you interested in pursuing a career doing something you loved earlier in your life, in an area you found interesting, and that you have a talent for? Complete Holland's *Career Interest Survey* and see what comes up.

Check out the careers that match your top three highest areas and discuss them with your parents or friends. It's helpful to have a fall-back position if your first choice does not work out.

Work relationships are best if they are respectful. Where bullying occurs then there should be steps that you can take to seek redress.

It is positive if you can be assertive with your work colleagues.

9. EMOTIONAL LIFE

Throughout this chapter you will find information about the positives and negatives of emotions. Read about how to manage emotions, and how to process them. Learn how to be happy in the present moment. There is discussion of a variety of positive and negative emotions, whether they are useful, and if they are not, how to let them go.

10. MENTAL HEALTH

If you or someone you know has issues with anxiety, depression, psychosis, eating disorders or phobias, then you may already have some knowledge and information about some of the points discussed here.

There is also information about possibilities for treatment. If you are not someone who has such issues then you may be thankful, and just take note of the section on happiness.

The rest of the chapter may be useful for your reference, should anyone you know have any of these issues.

11. ADDICTIONS

This chapter explores a number of addictions such as: tobacco, alcohol, prescription abuse, non-prescription drugs, pornography, gambling, social media, and gaming. There is also a general process of how to become free from your addiction, should you so desire.

12. SELF-ESTEEM

Everyone can read and discuss this chapter. If you have completed the core beliefs survey, downloadable from my website, then you will be able to note how high or low you have rated your self-esteem. See if you still rate it the same after reading through the characteristic behaviours of someone with low self-esteem.

Pick and choose how you might improve your self-esteem through some positive self-talk. You can work out what you could say to yourself that will counteract your negative self-talk.

13. ASSERTIVENESS

Read about the differences between passive, assertive, and aggressive behaviours. Work out where you are, and then you can work on becoming more assertive.

If you are passive then often the first step is to begin to say 'no' in some situations. Becoming assertive means that you are standing up for yourself, meeting your needs and taking others' needs into account as well. It takes some effort and practice, but it is possible to become assertive.

Even if you are often aggressive, you can learn to become assertive instead, so that you do not discount others' needs.

Practice with the use of "I Statements", by asking for help, and by saying no.

14. PERSONAL GROWTH

Hopefully, personal growth is something you aspire to.

Reading this chapter should get you into the frame of mind that enables you to think about what goals you'd like to set each year for your personal growth.

People usually like to feel that they are moving forward. Setting goals and taking action towards them can assist with the feeling of moving and progressing.

The incorporation of positive psychology exercises will benefit your emotional growth and also help your relationships. Make sure that you pay attention to your intuition as you go about your daily life.

Once you have read through all the chapters in the book, and have begun working through your issues to become the person you want to be, you will be well on your way to creating a life you'll love.

Personal change is an ongoing process, so the more consciously you work on yourself, the more you'll realise clarity and peace.

Be the best that you can be, and find your heart in your life!

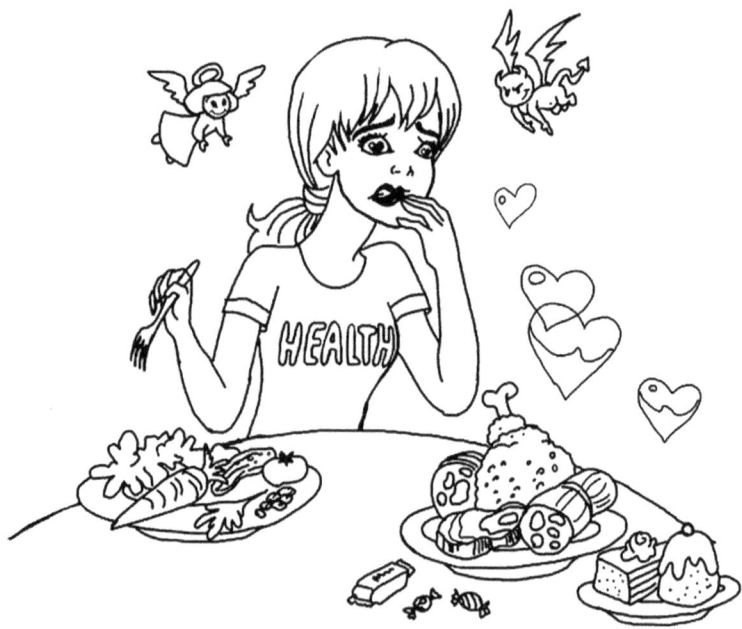

CHAPTER 2

PHYSICAL HEALTH

What does optimal health mean to you?

QUALITY OF LIFE

Physical health is an important aspect of wellbeing and quality of life. Wherever you are on the spectrum of health, from those who have chronic conditions or disabilities, through to those who are at the peak of physical fitness—everyone should regard their health as a priority.

The choices we make and the things we do always have consequences and some may have long-term effects. If you look after your body then you are giving yourself the greatest opportunities to be the best version of yourself that you can be.

Everything you put into your body will have an effect on you and your life, so it is always best to make an informed decision about the things you do.

One part of the body affects the whole.

Even the common cold causes most people to feel miserable.

The mind affects the body and the body affects the mind.

A physical therapy such as acupuncture will affect how you feel both in your body and in your mind.

A mental therapy such as cognitive behavioural therapy (CBT) can help how you feel in terms of mood, and this can have an impact on your behaviour.

As you feel better, you behave in different ways.

> Your body is fairly forgiving, but a good rule to follow is "everything in moderation". It is not true that if something is said to be good for you, then more is better.

PHYSICAL FACTORS AFFECTING HEALTH

From the moment of conception, your physical environment and the nutrition you receive have an effect on your health.

Early environments may pave the way for particular issues or problems later in life[1]. However, although you can't change the circumstances of your birth, as you grow up you can choose your behaviour to give yourself the best chances in life, by looking after yourself, having a well-balanced diet, exercising, and getting enough sleep[2]. Additionally, find the right environment for you—both internally and externally.

For instance, to protect yourself from future problems with skin cancer, use sunscreens with a high sun protection factor (SPF), wear a hat, and avoid sunbathing when the ultraviolet (UV) rays are at their strongest—between 10am and 4pm.

Skin cancer (melanoma) has a high incidence rate in Australia, and getting badly burnt—especially when young—increases the risk of skin cancer when older. This also goes for using tanning machines of any kind.

BRAIN POWER

In the simplest terms, your brain consists of three sections. The hindbrain (or reptilian brain), which governs survival instincts, the midbrain (or limbic system), which governs emotions and the frontal cortex (or neocortex), which governs thinking and reasoning.

Your brain is always monitoring your body and the information you are receiving from the outside world, and is constantly processing this information and predicting what may happen in case you need to take action.

You are the driver of your world. It is your brain that is communicating with every part of your body, and receiving information back too.

There are many neurons in your brain which form a network of connections to enable you to learn, remember, and to take in information from the outside world, process it, and respond. Your brain is a great prediction machine. It is always trying to predict what is going to happen next[3]. How it predicts what may happen is based on your past experiences, skills, knowledge and beliefs.

When you are young a lot of learning happens in a short space of time and the number of neurons in your brain becomes large, and many connections are being created between these neurons.

As you become older, a pruning process happens, which helps your brain to become more efficient. This pruning process reduces the number of connections between the neurons, so that only the more frequently used connections remain. This means that during childhood and young adulthood, if you engage in learning things that will stand you in good stead, particularly in the realms of critical thinking, reasoning and creativity, then working things out the "old-fashioned way"—by using your brain rather than just relying on technology to do the short cuts for you—will be better for you in the long term.

There is evidence that the use of technology[4] is having a detrimental effect on people's ability to be creative, to write, to think critically, and to use reasoning in ways that enhance their lives[5]. This may be one of the reasons why young people's mental health has been declining over time[6].

GUT HEALTH

In recent years, the importance of gut health on both the body and mind has come into prominence. The complex interaction between the microbiome (the gut environment with the different bacteria) and diet, and how this affects health across many different conditions has been at the heart of some research.

Evidence is coming to light to indicate that our microbiome and physical environment (including our diet and lifestyle) may be at the root of many illnesses and diseases[7]. Thus, diet is very important.

By changing what you put inside your body, you can improve or reduce the percentage of good microbiota (bacteria) in your gut. For instance, connections are now being made between the microbiome and autoimmune diseases including Parkinsons[8], multiple sclerosis, and other kinds of conditions such as coeliac disease[9].

So, what can you do to help ensure your physical health is the best it can be?

Everybody is different, so you may need to take a little time working out what is right for your biology and physiology—and some of those things may change at different points in your life—but by and large there are some basic rules that you can follow.

Firstly, if you have a course of antibiotics, ensure that you follow up or take concurrently a good probiotic to replace the good bacteria in your gut[10].

Secondly, diet is particularly important because it does affect your nutrition and microbiome[11],[12]. Thirdly, the reduction and elimination of toxins is also important. Particular foods may cause inflammation that can impact your overall wellbeing over time. What you feed your body can cause your microbiome to favour one lot of microbiotas over others (there are many different families of microbiota and some are more conducive for wellbeing than others). What this means is that eventually you may become less healthy on a number of levels, including mentally.

It is a fact that we have neurons in a number of areas in our body—not just in our brain. There are neurons in our hearts, and neurons in our guts.

The vagus nerve is the pathway that carries messages between our guts and brains[13].

In our bodies, the autonomic nervous system (that operates the unconscious processes in our body) and the central nervous systems (brain and spinal cord) work together. The vagus nerve is one of 12 cranial nerves (they are in pairs) in our body, and as part of the autonomic nervous system (ANS) is responsible for digestion, heart rate, breathing, and other unconscious processes, such as reflex actions. It is the longest nerve in our body and runs from the brain stem to the colon[14], and has links with the face muscles, heart, and other abdominal organs. It is also a two-way information highway. There are a number of different means of transport that these messages may take, but there is certainly traffic both ways[15].

A recent and popular theory about the function of this nerve and what it might mean for treatment is contained in the Polyvagal Theory. The Polyvagal Theory[16] explains how our body's nervous system affects our social behaviour, emotions, and stress responses. It suggests that there are three parts to our nervous system: one for social engagement and connection, one for fight-or-flight responses to danger, and one for shutdown or freeze responses, and that these systems have evolved with us as we became social creatures. These are all interconnected and work together. Our ability to switch between them helps us adapt to different situations. The theory highlights the importance of social cues and experiences in shaping our physiological reactions and overall well-being.

Since messages and information go both ways between your guts and your brain, this means that what you put in your body really does affect your brain: and thus, your mental state and emotional wellbeing. Additionally, the vagus nerve acts as a counterpoint to stress. So, through activities like yoga, meditating, and breathing, you can utilise the vagus nerve pathway to reduce the amount of stress you are feeling. One point to note is that the theory details are not necessarily proven as yet, and there is some opposition to the total package[17]. However, this does not mean that the particular aspects for treatment are not working in some way – it does not make the effects wrong, if the particular pathway to those effects are different in theory.

One effective breathing exercise is to breathe in for the count of 4, hold for 2, and then breathe out for the count of 6, expelling all the air from the bottom of your lungs. This exercise is also helpful with getting to sleep.

THE SOCIAL CONTEXT

Consider the broader context when exploring what your choices could be in determining how you behave and what you are eating, drinking or accepting into your body and immediate environment.

As consumers, even if we trust the government and corporations to act in our best interests, it may be better to take responsibility for making our own decisions about what we eat and how we organise our lifestyle and routines. We do have this responsibility in any case.

While it may be essential to live harmoniously with others and to accept the rules, taking personal responsibility for health choices is advisable. Genetics, environment, and social factors can affect health outcomes. Focus on controlling what you consume, making informed decisions, and listening to your body's needs to improve overall well-being. Once you are taking control of what you can control, then you will know that you have been doing your best to look after yourself. Many things may happen that are both unexpected and outside of your domain of control. You are not the cause of everything that happens to you. Sometimes physical disease and illness arise from social factors, genetics, and environmental factors.

By paying more attention to your body and what it might be telling you from any symptoms, and being aware of choosing the things your body likes (which may be different from the things *you* like), you may begin to feel more positive about yourself.

FOOD FOR THOUGHT

DIET

Everyone's physiology may vary depending on many factors including genetic, and environmental. What you put into your body physically forms the foundation of your current internal environment which affects the nutrients your body is able to extract, and what it can do with them.

Are your food choices relatively healthy, or are the things you eat not very good for you? Are you eating the right amount?

Eating too much or too little can be damaging to your body. You can find out more about eating disorders in Chapter 10.

Whatever you eat, chew it well. There is some evidence[18] that the more you chew your food, the fuller you feel, which means you are likely to eat less. Chewing each mouthful thirty times rather than fifteen (which is usual) will assist with this.

If you were ever told to chew your food instead of wolfing it down, you were given good advice.

Most authorities now recommend eating food closest to its natural state. Some foods need cooking, some may be more nutritious raw (such as capsicum, lettuce, celery, cucumber) but the fewer additives and processes added to food, the better. It is widely recognised that processed meat in large quantities causes a higher risk of cancer. Therefore, you could limit the amount of ham, bacon, sausages, salami, and other processed meats you eat to reduce this risk[19].

Additionally, what is now called "ultra-processed food", which is essentially fast food, take-away food, and meals and foods you can buy in packages, are unhealthy and can cause long-term health problems, including heart disease, diabetes, and cancer[20].

This is mostly because the amounts of sugar, salt, and fats that are added have been worked out in the ratio that is addictive for the reward systems in our brains.

The advertising and marketing around these foods is pervasive and persuasive.

It is therefore important for you to foster a sense of choosing your own menu from fresh foods that you purchase and prepare for yourself. In this way, you will be missing out on huge amounts of sugar, salt, and bad fats that are added to processed and pre-prepared foods—and your body will thank you.

Vegetables should be as fresh as possible. Some people prefer organic vegetables and fruit. There are more shops and greater access allowing for this option now than ever before, although it does depend where you live. Frozen vegetables are fine although some may need some care if you are freezing them yourself. Generally, bought frozen vegetables and fruit should be fine. It is always better not to refreeze food once unfrozen, particularly meat. A variety of food is usually a good idea where possible, and limiting your meat intake to a few times per week may be healthier.

By including some meals of fresh fish, you will also be getting some Omega 3. Generally, processed food and junk food should be eaten only rarely.

IDEAS AND BELIEFS

We eat for sustenance and energy, but meals can often have a social element too.

As a result of this, food and drink have become laden with ideas and beliefs around cultural and social situations. Eating meals together can be a bonding experience and this can make a positive contribution to our wellbeing.

Eating may also have a moral and ethical element. Some people choose to be vegetarians because they have a belief that killing animals for consumption is wrong. There may also be concerns over the methods of killing, or the fear and suffering that the animals feel.

Food choices can also be made over farming methods and ethical practices. Additionally, there can be concerns over the amount of energy that may be involved in the production and transportation of the food.

More consumers are now ascribing to the idea of buying local, and of choosing plant-based products over animal products. Reducing animal consumption can be helpful for the environment.

Generally speaking, the larger the animal, the greater the amount of carbon, water and energy used in the production of the meat. This means that cattle are high on the list, sheep are lower, and chickens are lower still.

Choosing to eat less meat and more plant-based food is therefore healthier for you and better for the planet.

Where you have a belief that any sentient being and products deriving from sentient beings should not be consumed, the most usual choice is veganism.

Vegans do not eat any kind of animal or animal product, which includes dairy and eggs. This reflects a philosophy that rejects the commodity status of animals and the exploitation of them for human consumption[21]. Sometimes people find that choosing a vegan diet suits their body better.

It is an individual choice to be a vegetarian or vegan, as it is to follow any kind of diet. However, whatever diet you choose, it is important to ensure that you are getting all the nutrients you require.

If you have dietary restrictions, supplements or some other ways of fortifying your food intake may be necessary to ensure a balanced diet.

Investigation and planning are a good idea.

THE APPLICATION OF SCIENCE

The best diets are those backed by science. The Mediterranean Diet and the CSIRO Wellbeing Diet are cases in point.

Studies that have been carried out on various diets appear to show that the best diet to feed yourself is the Mediterranean Diet. This is a diet that is rich in fruit and vegetables, legumes, whole grains, nuts, olive oil, fish, and low in red meat and sugar.

The benefits of this diet have been shown to alleviate depression[22], to improve longevity and cardiovascular health, and to reduce the risk of diabetes[23].

The CSIRO Wellbeing Diet was devised by the CSIRO scientists in Australia[24]. It is based on healthy food and reduced carbohydrates. Small portions are a feature of this diet.

FOOD FAD DIETS

Over time, different diets may be in vogue.

Sometimes the diets may have good aspects to them, but they may not be helpful overall.

A lot of fad diets may help you to lose weight over a certain period of time, but not be good over the long-term. Keep this in mind if trying out a fad diet. It's a good idea to scrutinise the levels of nutrition in the diet and to ensure that you are meeting all your nutritional needs.

THE FOOD PYRAMID

The Healthy Eating Food Pyramid[25] refers to the recommended food groups, and was updated in 2013. It is relatively flexible and allows foods to be eaten from all food groups, focusing on whole foods rather than nutrients.

It suggests 70% of our intake should be from unprocessed plant foods: vegetables, legumes, and fruit; along with a moderate amount of dairy, meat, seafood, and eggs; including a small serve of healthy fats per day; and limiting added sugar and salt. As far as drinking goes, water is the best choice. The recommendation is to reduce or cut out sugary drinks. It is also advisable to cut out energy drinks, which contain a lot of sugar and caffeine.

It is still recommended to eat five serves of vegetables and two serves of fruit a day. This shows that fruit and vegetables should be a major part of your diet.

Eating a balanced diet that includes the recommended food groups and only rarely eating junk food or ultra-processed food will mean that you are doing well.

To form good eating habits, home cooked meals are best. Ensure that you wash what you eat, whether you cook it or not. Non-organic food may be grown with pesticides—and would you really want to ingest these, when they are often carcinogenic?

You can make tasty, cheap meals from scratch fairly quickly, and even though some meals may take longer to prepare, the reward is in knowing they are better for you than junk food, and that your friends or family can meet together around the table to eat. This helps communication and enhances your relationships.

SLEEP

It is also important for your health to get enough sleep. Sleep allows you to process the previous day's events, refreshing both the mind and body. You should be getting about seven to eight hours sleep a night. If you are getting less then you are probably operating at less than 100%. Tiredness can lead to bad judgements, memory issues, stress, and long-term health issues. Get into a routine of winding down before you go to bed[26].

Melanin helps us get to sleep, and you can train your brain to get into the production of melanin earlier in the evening by turning off bright artificial lights for a few hours before you go to bed.

You can also purchase blue UV light blocking glasses, or set options on your phone and TV to adjust the lighting to night-time settings.

The blue light emitted by screens wakes up your brain, and this means that it is much more difficult to get to sleep.

For this reason, it is recommended to stop using phones and computer screens for at least an hour before going to bed.

Going outside for a walk or to water the garden in the early morning sunshine or daylight shortly after you get up is also beneficial, and can help reset your circadian rhythm (your body clock) so that you may get to sleep more easily[27].

Getting enough sleep is crucial to good health.

Getting either too little sleep or too much may both be detrimental in the long term. Sleeping more than ten hours a night may lead to high blood sugar and diabetes. Oversleeping is also linked to negative thinking and depression. Since over-sleepers move less, there is the likelihood of obesity. Additionally, there is an increased risk of cardiovascular disease, for women as opposed to men[28].

On the other hand, too little sleep has been linked to tiredness, making mistakes, poor decision-making, confusion, and, if lack of sleep occurs over time consistently (6 hours or less) then this has the same effect on concentrating and driving ability as having a blood alcohol level of .05.[29]

Something to note is that it is not just sleep that is important, but rest.

If you feel that you cannot think straight, this is your brain protecting itself.

This is the time you need to rest. Do something completely different, go for a walk, go and get together with a friend, read, or even do nothing. You cannot expect your brain to work perfectly for you 100% of the time without a break.

Rest is even more important if you are not getting all the sleep you require. It is within our sleep cycles that the brain is restored, toxins cleaned out, and memories consolidated. Give yourself these benefits, and ultimately your brain and your body will work better for you.

From your teens to young adulthood, your circadian rhythms change to later times. What this means is that it is not your fault if you find you're not in synch with your school hours. It is your body adjusting to the stage of life you are at[30]. There has been some talk about changing school hours—particularly in high school, due to this factor. It is not easy to learn if you are exhausted all the time.

TIPS

- Buy wholemeal or wholegrain bread instead of white bread

- Sourdough bread may be healthier for you

- Reduce or cut ultra-processed foods

- Reduce your sugar intake

- Home-cook your meals

- Drink more water – perhaps up to 2 litres over the day – not all at once.

- Reduce or cut out sugary drinks

- Cut out energy drinks – too much caffeine and sugar cause dental problems

---

- Follow the healthy food pyramid or the Mediterranean diet
- Eat sensible portion sizes – have smaller portions to lose weight
- Chew your mouthfuls for longer
- Get enough sleep and rest, as well as giving yourself breaks
- Keep moving, rather than sitting down for extended periods of time

WEIGHT

We all enjoy life more when we can be healthy and well. It is a great deal better overall to have your body in a healthy weight category since this means that you are less likely to suffer from ill health complications. However, if you are overweight it is not the end of the world.

Although your body is part of you, you are not just your body.

There are more aspects to you than just what people see the first time they meet you. While advertising and social media place a lot of importance on appearance, it does not define who you are. Who you are as a person is so much more important.

See the chapter on self-esteem for more ideas on this.

Your body has an idea of the weight you should be.

This occurs over time. There are multiple factors that feed into your adult body weight, including genetics, childhood nutrition and environment, eating habits, cultural, lifestyle, disability, mental health, and many other things such as availability and convenience[31].

Relating to the idea that the body has an idea of your ideal weight, was shown through a small experiment carried out by Michael Moseley in which an increased food intake for people who were normally lean over a period of four weeks.

This group put on a bit of weight, but not as much as expected, and they lost it again fairly quickly after the experiment ended. This also works the other way.

If obese people lose weight, then unless they really change their eating habits and lifestyle in order to change the body's idea of the weight it should be, then the weight will just go back on[32].

One point to note is that it is far better to be fit and fat, than unfit. They do not cancel each other out.

KYLIE'S STORY

When Kylie was twenty-five, she was nearly 100kgs and had very high blood pressure. She got read the riot act by her doctor. He said if she didn't change her lifestyle then she'd go to an early grave. This was a wake-up call. Her response was to change her diet, and to replace happy hour with walking. She lost 30kgs in eight months. She got fit. She recently ran in a half-marathon, and has never been healthier in her life.

The percentage of obese people in our society is increasing. The use of fats and sugars in shop-bought foods (which are usually ultra-processed) probably plays a major part in this, as well as poor dietary habits. Childhood diet may have a role too, by giving the body the ideal weight concept and habits that can be difficult to break.

While a weight-loss diet may help people to slim down in the short-term, unless there are lifestyle changes and long-term changes in dietary habits and mindset, the weight just goes back on.

There is now evidence that the reason for this is that hormones in the body cause the person to feel hungry. In order to make long-lasting changes you can start making healthy decisions[33]. Becoming fit is a good goal and a great achievement, but exercise by itself may not be enough to help you lose weight. You may need to change what you eat, when you eat, and how much you eat.

Cutting right back on fast foods will help, or even cutting them out altogether, if possible. Making small changes over time in the food you are eating is the best plan. Particularly start to eat more vegetables, and continuing to add more until you are eating mostly vegetables. Sometimes we may be hungry due to our body wanting some particular nutrient. So, you can slowly change to eating vegetables and fruit and this is much more likely to help you slowly lose weight, which is much better for you than otherwise[34]. At the same time, ensure you are getting enough protein too.

Home-cooked meals may require some extra planning and take a up a little more of your time, but improving your diet and nutrition should provide you with extra energy, meaning you can get more done with less effort, so things should soon balance out.

If you put yourself on a program to lose weight it is important to address your mindset, as well as your diet and exercise regime.

If you monitor your physical weight then you could also monitor your psychological wellbeing.

This can be done with the help of a psychologist or NLP Practitioner.

NLP stands for neuro-linguistic programming, and it may be helpful in the process of weight loss, as it helps the conscious mind and the unconscious mind to align, so that automatic behaviour may be changed. This can make achieving your goals a lot easier than just using will power. A mindset coach may also be helpful here. You could even put your own weight-loss program into place with the help of my first book *A Practical Guide for Self Change 35*.

ONE POPULAR WAY TO LOSE WEIGHT

Intermittent fasting, or the 5:2 diet, was made popular by Michael Moseley[36].

With the 5:2 diet, you eat normally for five days in the week, and choose two days in which you restrict your calorie intake to 600 calories.

There is some evidence that this diet works and helps those who are overweight to lose weight, as well as reducing disease markers in the form of lowering cholesterol, blood pressure, and blood sugar[37].

If you also start choosing to eat a greater proportion of healthy food and less junk food then you may find extra benefits and improvements in your general health too. This diet helps weight to drop slowly, which is much better for your body than losing it rapidly, and makes it more likely you will keep the weight off, provided you make some lifestyle changes.

Another variation of this intermittent fasting regime is called the 16:8 diet, where you eat within an 8-hour period during the day. For instance, having breakfast at 11am, and finishing dinner around 7pm, with no food between 7pm and 11am the next day, which means you are fasting for 16 hours.

Your routine and lifestyle habits will play a part in whether this will work for you.

If it does, then it could be a good option.

However, make sure you consult with your medical practitioner before embarking on a diet involving intermittent fasting, since there are circumstances in which fasting may be dangerous to your health.

There is recent evidence that eating within a range of around nine hours resets your body and circadian rhythms, so this could be an added benefit to engaging in this diet, at least for a while[38].

DIETARY RESTRICTIONS

Having dietary restrictions, allergies or sensitivities may be difficult, especially when socialising and going out for meals.

The situation may be easier when only one or two foods need to be avoided, but if there are a number of foods then it may become more complicated.

When it comes down to quality of life, and a matter of health and wellness, considerations around how to manage dietary restrictions is obviously important. Decisions can be made with such things in mind.

You may need help, support and understanding from friends, family, and professionals, to ensure you are able to get the most out of your social life, in spite of the restrictions you face. Your doctor or health practitioner should be able to advise you of resources that can offer you help and support. In some areas, there are more dietary options available now than there have been in the past.

Seek out the restaurants and cafés that provide the foods that meet your needs.

Again, by making your meals at home, you can ensure you are eating the right foods for you.

SUPPLEMENTS

Should you take supplements? Vitamins and dietary supplements are big business.

There is a reasonable weight of evidence that if you have a varied and healthy diet then supplements may well be a waste of time and money[39].

Exceptions to this appear to include Omega 3 and vitamin D, and pregnant women should also take folate, iron, and iodine (which is in iodised salt).

It may even be helpful to start taking these before pregnancy. However, with Omega 3, eating oily fish is probably better than taking a supplement. A recent study of Omega 3 supplements on the market in Hong Kong found that a large proportion contained carcinogenic toxins[40]. Whether similar proportions would also be applicable in Australia or in other countries could be reasonably possible.

So, sourcing your Omega 3 from food is likely to be more beneficial than taking supplements. However, because our bodies do not make Omega 3s, if you find it difficult to get enough Omega 3 in your diet, seek out good quality sources for the supplement.

Hemp oil may be one option. If you aren't eating the foods, or you are deficient in the nutrients in spite of eating food rich in Omega 3s, then supplements may be the best way to go.

The safest supplements are likely to be the ones that many people commonly require, and that have stood over the test of time.

These include calcium, vitamin D, vitamin B and vitamin C.

Even with these, unless you have been assessed by a health professional who has determined that you have a deficiency, or you have specific conditions or circumstances that require supplements, then food is likely to be the best way to get the correct nutrition.

It is also better not to mix a lot of supplements together, as interactions may occur and you may end up in a worse condition than when you started[41], such as with an increased risk of cancer.

Be cautious of popular hype when it comes to supplements.

For instance, curcumin is now all the rage. Curcumin is a major component of turmeric, which has also become very popular in recent years. However, a recent study has shown that continued ingestion of curcumin causes liver damage[42].

Therefore, unless you have specific conditions where you need curcumin, or any other preparation, the best practice is to use such supplements only until your body is better.

Things that are usually spices, or used sparingly (such as poppy seeds) are probably best kept to small amounts. Poppy seeds in large amounts have also been shown to damage your body[43]. If you are healthy already, taking supplements may not make you healthier, but may instead cause problems.

Reading the labels on supplement bottles and also on any food packaging is strongly advised. This is quite difficult to navigate at times however, and it could be that by adopting a policy of fresh and home-cooked food for the majority of meals, as you will be able to navigate your choices more easily.

After all, it's far easier to know what's in a fresh potato than in a potato chip.

It might be helpful to have Omega 3 if you have rheumatoid arthritis. Studies have shown inconclusive results for any other benefits. It might also be helpful to have vitamin C if you smoke and vitamin B if you are stressed.

Some people may be low in vitamin D, and this can be helped through supplements or a daily dose of sunlight. You only need about 10 to 30 minutes of bright sunlight a few times a week to maintain healthy blood levels of vitamin D. The lighter your skin, the less time it takes.

If you are interested in finding out more about supplements and feel that they may be of benefit to, you could discuss your situation with your doctor. You may also have a blood test and see what your doctor recommends.

Supplements may also be taken for muscle gain. Preparations containing protein, vitamins, and minerals may help this process. These need to be taken at the same time as working out. However, it depends on the results you want. You may choose to eat a healthy diet without taking supplements, which is the best option. While being strong can be a great goal, it is quite possible to be strong without having huge muscles, and it is always good to keep everything in balance.

ALTERNATIVE TREATMENTS

There are a number of alternative options to explore if you are not having any luck with conventional medicine. There are more branches of alternative medicine in functional or integrative medicine. These branches of alternative medicine consider and treat the whole person, rather than just the symptoms of a physical condition.

Other options in the field of alternative practitioners include nutritionists, naturopaths and acupuncturists. With some research and exploration, you may be able to find the modalities and practitioners that work for you. An osteopath may also be a good alternative to a chiropractor for skeletal issues and soft tissue problems.

It is important to be aware that just because herbal medications and preparations do not claim to be drugs that they have no effect on the system. Herbal medications and preparations still contain chemicals, and there are many herbs that interact with prescription drugs. If you are taking any prescription medications, check with your medical doctor to see if any herbs you are considering taking are safe for you to use and do not interact with your prescription medication.

DISABILITIES

No matter what type of disability you have, you are a normal person managing life the best you can.

If you are a carer, you have the exceptionally important job of supporting your loved one or client.

When you have a disability, there may be specific services and needs that you have which, if fulfilled, will enable you to gain optimal functioning and wellbeing.

With the National Disability Insurance Scheme in Australia (NDIS), it is to be hoped that those needing help will find positive benefits when issues with the scheme are resolved, so all those who need help actually get it and greater inclusivity becomes the status quo.

Everyone deserves respect and understanding, and social inclusion is an important concept for society to engage with on all levels.

While you may be restricted in some ways, you still have the potential to live your best life.

Your beliefs about yourself can have a big impact on your world. By giving yourself every opportunity to look after your physical health and wellbeing, you give yourself the best opportunity to reach, and remain, at the top of your game.

CHRONIC CONDITIONS

Whatever chronic condition you have, whether an autoimmune disease, chronic pain, or other disease or disorder, then you are no doubt attempting to manage it in the best way you can.

It may take many trips to the doctor or specialist before you find something that helps your condition or allows you to be in the best space possible. Your health is likely to be a major concern and priority.

If you have good days and bad days then work towards having more good days.

If there is anything you can do to make more good days, then do it.

Sometimes the impact of your condition may seem a bit unpredictable, and so it's important to be compassionate with yourself at all times.

You may be on many medications and be at risk of addiction to painkillers.

Where you have a good support network, you will be in a better position than someone who is isolated. Work on your friendships and family relationships in a positive manner to ensure you have the support you need.

It is important to ask questions of your medical team. Be assertive, ask for information, and question them about how they came to suggest specific things.

Question the side effects of medications and make sure you are on the best ones for you. Medication only reduces symptoms; it is not a cure.

Different medications have varying effects on individuals, even when they are in the same family of medications.

Ensure you are on the best medication with the least side effects to control your specific symptoms.

RECENT TRENDS

In recent times there has been a rise in autoimmune disease, food intolerances, and allergies in the Western World. An inflammatory response occurs when the immune system's natural response to an external threat—whether bacteria or virus—is triggered, but there is no real threat. The body can, over time, develop a chronic low-grade inflammation. You may or may not notice symptoms.

Symptoms may arise in autoimmune diseases, food intolerances, or allergies.

In autoimmune diseases such as arthritis, multiple sclerosis, lupus, type 1 diabetes, Graves' Disease, and inflammatory bowel disease, the body is already primed and has a chronic inflammatory response. Eating foods that cause inflammation may exacerbate the condition. Eating foods that are anti-inflammatory may be of benefit both in the short-term and long-term.

Essentially, if you are looking after your microbiome and feeding yourself healthy food and have a relatively healthy lifestyle, getting the right amount of everything, then you are doing your best.

Food allergies and food intolerances are different. The difference is that a food allergy sparks off the immune system to create a kind of reaction that may be mild to life threatening (anaphylactic shock).

An allergy is a response from the body to usually normally tolerated foods. A food intolerance or sensitivity on the other hand causes the body to react in a chemical response to the particular food or drink. It is not the immune system reacting[44].

However, food sensitivities, intolerances and allergies can lead to chronic low-grade inflammation. Allergies do not necessarily cause an anaphylactic response that is life threatening. When they do cause an anaphylactic response, a shot of adrenaline is necessary.

Other responses and reactions may require changes to your diet.

For example, when I was young, I was allergic to cow's milk and egg white, and the reaction to these foods was that I developed eczema.

It took many years for the eczema to disappear completely. Over time, I became less allergic to these foods—or at least I thought I did.

There is now more research being conducted on chronic inflammation and some gathering evidence that even just eating some foods your body is sensitive to, or slightly intolerant of, can lead to chronic inflammation. This can lead to illnesses that may be difficult to treat, such as autoimmune disorders, mental health conditions including depression, and irritable bowel syndrome (which can be caused purely by psychological stress)[45].

Much evidence is showing that going on the Mediterranean diet is beneficial for specific mental health conditions such as depression, anxiety and stress, as well as for general health and wellbeing as previously discussed[46].

If you have some symptoms and you suspect that you might have a food intolerance, then there is something that you can do about it.

A doctor or a naturopath may be helpful in defining the problem. Otherwise having a proper allergy testing would be appropriate.

Alternatively, you can take yourself off the particular food you think may be causing a reaction for two to four weeks. At the end of this time, you reintroduce the food and make a note of the effects and any symptoms you get. Compare how you felt during the time you were off the food and how you feel being back on it. If there is no discernible difference, then perhaps the food is ok for you.

Another possibility is to find a reputable company who will test your unique body sensitivities. The degree to which results may be relatively correct could be tested through the above method of food elimination—possibly for months rather than weeks.

One thing to know is that as we age, our bodies may need different nutrients and our digestive system may change.

Sometimes, it becomes less able to absorb nutrients. It is important to go to your doctor when you perceive changes in your body, no matter what kind of changes.

This doesn't mean that you are running for help every time you get a slight difference in your functioning, but it does mean that if you have noticed a consistent change for about a month or so (depending on the symptoms and effects on your life) then rather than treating it yourself, go and check it out with a medical professional.

While Google can be helpful, it is not a diagnostic tool and a real person with a medical degree is required.

When we are young, our bodies are more able to process what we are eating, and we can probably go a bit harder than when we are older. There is, however, a case for starting early in treating your body well. Since ultra-processed foods and foods high in sugar have been widely available people become unhealthier and there has been a greater incidence of illnesses related to inflammation.

It is also the case that some illnesses can strike us at any time, and so finding a good, empathic doctor who will explain things to you and with whom you have a positive relationship is key.

FOODS MORE LIKELY TO CAUSE AN INFLAMMATORY RESPONSE

Dairy, meat from grain-fed animals, processed/cured meats, alcohol, vegetable oils, artificial sweeteners, sugar, refined grains such as white flour and rice, trans fats, saturated fats[47],[48].

ANTI-INFLAMMATORY FOODS

Olive oil, green leafy vegetables, nuts, fatty fish, fruit including berries, tomatoes, garlic and onions, herbs and spices[49].

While nuts are very good for you, it is also the case that in moderation is best. Keep to one handful per day. Too many nuts may cause diarrhoea.

SELF-HEALING

Evidence is gathering that people can heal themselves through the power of belief and the power of the mind.

The placebo effect has been known for a long time, and is taken into account in studies researching the effectiveness of medication. As Dr Joe Dispenza suggests, 'you are the placebo'[50].

Self-healing is not necessarily a cure. It may, however, allow you to get to a much better place, and may alleviate some symptoms.

It very much depends upon individual circumstances and individual responses.

Some conditions are also more amenable to self-healing than others. Although it seems that some people manage what can be seen as a miracle, because it is the power of the mind that helps, the best way to effect self-healing is to work on your unconscious mind[51].

Where you are interested in healing yourself from some kind of health condition, it could be beneficial to explore all levels of your being. Thus, external factors may play a role, including what you are eating and drinking, as well what is in your internal environment. Your internal environment includes your mind, your values, your beliefs, and how all these aspects connect. Stress may be a factor, sleep may be a factor, and your life situation may be a factor.

Your lifestyle is another area that requires investigation. These different aspects make up "you-being-in-the-world".

See it as a holistic assessment. One thing to know is that while everything affects everything else, sometimes what occurs is just on a physical level, and nothing else will work except conventional medicine.

Where you have an obvious physical symptom, it can be helpful to have it checked medically. It can be very easy to ignore symptoms or to put them down to various things that you may think of, and assume they are nothing.

If you tend to be fearful of health issues, then this may mean you are reading things into normal body functioning that may not actually be there. It is important to make this distinction, between not paying attention, or assuming too much.

Essentially it is best to pay attention to your body, but in an overall view rather than a minute and detailed view.

EXERCISE

Exercise is activity requiring physical effort, carried out to maintain or improve health and fitness.

Among the different activities that provide exercise, there are possibilities to exercise alone or in groups. You can also engage in exercise individually but among others, such as in a gym. There is an abundance of choice of exercise, and which forms of exercise you choose comes down to your decisions about what works for you.

The World Health Organisation[52] recommends that adults aged between 18 and 64 engage in at least 150 - 300 minutes of moderate exercise each week. This exercise should include both muscle strengthening and aerobic exercise at least three times a week. An alternative is to do at least 75 minutes of vigorous intensity aerobic physical activity throughout the week. For the best results, you should increase moderate intensity physical activity to 300 minutes per week or vigorous aerobic physical activity 150 minutes per week. They also suggest limiting the amount of sedentary time. They strongly recommend for everyone to do more than the recommended amounts of activity, due to the highly detrimental effects of sitting for long periods of time.

WHAT'S IN IT FOR ME?

There are numerous benefits to taking regular exercise.

Many studies have shown that exercise improves cardiorespiratory and muscular fitness, and helps bone health. Additionally, those who are more active have lower rates of coronary heart disease, high blood pressure, stroke, type 2 diabetes, metabolic syndrome, colon and breast cancer, and depression. There is also less risk of hip fracture or vertebral fracture, and more likelihood of achieving weight maintenance and having a healthier body mass index (BMI)[53].

Regular exercise also improves chronic conditions and cognitive function.

All in all, it makes good sense to exercise on a regular basis. However, ensure that you are not overdoing it. Moderation is good here too. There may be external pressures from society and loved ones, or internal expectations on yourself due to your beliefs around what is best in terms of exercise.

HEALTH BENEFITS

The effect of exercise is, to some extent, an individual response.

It appears that there may be a small percentage of people who do not respond to exercise by losing weight[54]. This group still get the other health benefits of exercise, so there is no reason to despair if you seem to be in this small category. You can still exercise for fitness and look at making dietary changes to help support weight loss.

Studies have also been done on life expectancy and a sedentary lifestyle—results show that those with a sedentary lifestyle are at risk of dying earlier than those who exercise more[55]. These are some good reasons to get into exercise!

RECENT TRENDS IN EXERCISE

Exercise is becoming more a proactive and preventative effort, rather than tacked on when possible.

Yoga and Pilates are popular, with yoga having had more research applied.

Findings of the benefits of practising yoga are strong for both men and women. Additionally, it has been shown that the use of high intensity interval training (HIIT) has a similar effect to more exercise hours. In this, you exercise as hard as you can go for 1 minute at a time, then rest for one minute, and repeat the process.

High intensity interval training can be almost as good as exercising for longer periods of time[56].

One particular routine to do consists of five minutes exercise three times a week. This involves doing a small warm up first, then:

- One minute of star jumps, as quickly as possible
- Rest for one minute
- One minute of squats, as quickly as possible
- Rest for one minute
- One minute of sprinting on the spot, as quickly as possible
- Rest for one minute
- Then, depending on your capacity, you can do more exercises for a span of one minute, adding on to this base. However, three to four repetitions are optimal.
- The particular exercises you do need to be based on your own current level of fitness and physical comfort. Go easy on your body. Start small and work your way up as your fitness and strength levels improve.
- You can repeat the same exercise, such as running on the spot.

You can do this routine at home. It will cost you no money and it will improve your fitness.

WHAT REALLY HELPS IN EXERCISE

When we exercise, there are multiple functions happening in our body that means that we improve our body functioning overall.

By moving our muscles, and limbs, we improve circulation to all of our organs, not just our muscles. Improved circulation helps the heart, and improves endurance[57].

The immune system improves and any kind of recovery that is needed is enhanced.

It also gives a general strengthening to all of the body systems.

Breathing is improved, as is lung function overall.

Often when we are engaging in exercise, we are outside.

This is where there are plants, nature, and fresh air which can be good for improving your mental clarity and feelings of connection to the world.

Different types of exercise are available and it can be best to do those that you are drawn to. Even just walking is really good[58] for heart health, overall health and wellbeing (and for some cancers, osteoporosis and diabetes).

After exercise you are likely to have a more refreshing sleep and fall asleep faster than otherwise.

During exercise, the brain releases a number of chemicals that then are sent to various parts of your body. When you do vigorous exercise, the brain generally releases endorphins. These tend to give you a slight high, or feeling of wellbeing.

You feel invigorated and energised.

Exercise is very helpful in many different health recovery situations, including managing difficult treatments such as chemotherapy, and more generally in relation to any recovery from illness such as a heart attack.

This does not mean that you go running around, but walking and moving rather than sitting down all the time are good for you[59].

Exercise is also an anti-aging practice and keeps you supple, flexible, younger and more able to improve your immune system functioning so you may not get as ill and remain healthier longer[60].

MAKING CHANGES

As you go about your day, you can make changes that will help you to be fitter. You could use the stairs instead of the lift, and walk or cycle rather than driving, if the journey is not too far. It all adds up.

Exercise doesn't necessarily have to take large blocks of time or take you away from your daily routines. Even housework provides moderate exercise.

If you play a sport then you are probably getting the right amount of exercise in your week. Whether you participate in a sport or attend an exercise class you are making good, healthy choices that will be beneficial in the long term.

TIPS

- Take the stairs when you can
- Walk for 30 minutes a day – this doesn't have to be all at once
- Go cycling when you can
- Book into an exercise class – we are more motivated when others are involved
- Remember that every little bit of exercise adds up
- Play a sport of some kind

- Make an exercise plan and stick with it
- Best all-round exercises include dancing, cycling, and walking
- If you are also in a group of people and singing, this is one of the best for wellbeing

MAKING DECISIONS

It will be easier to make good decisions if you have your health as a top priority.

It is a value that you can make important.

When you need to make decisions about what you eat or drink, then you can ask yourself the question, 'Is this part of a balanced diet?'

Such decisions need to be made at the time you can influence the outcome, so when you are making a shopping list, when you're shopping or when you're in a café, bar or restaurant.

The same applies to exercise—do you really need to take the bus or the car, or could you walk or cycle instead? It's important to look at the long-term benefits rather than merely the short-term emotions or convenience. Keep your health high on your agenda and make informed decisions.

Even small changes such as walking to the local shops instead of taking the car or bus, or eating whole grains, such as wholemeal bread or brown rice rather than white bread or white rice, will be beneficial. Making healthy decisions means that you are acting in the present for your future.

Physical health is not just in your body, it is in your mind too, and in your whole external environment— we are affected by what is happening in the world, our families, and our social circle.

All these things affect our health. Since we are only in control of ourselves, it becomes important for us to take responsibility for our health and wellbeing. We can mitigate and reduce some of the stress we may feel about particular topics and our place in the world.

Some of the ways that we can do this will be discussed later.

LOOKING AFTER YOUR FIVE SENSES

We humans have five senses through which we receive information from the outside world into our brains. These are: sight, hearing, touch, taste, and smell.

It is helpful to consider looking after these senses carefully as you go through life. What this means is that if there are recommendations to wear protective clothing or similar items for work or other activities, then do this.

If you have good eyesight to start with, then maintain your sight where possible.

If you have good hearing, then it is also important to protect this. Loud noise, whether at work, at concerts, or through headphones and ear buds can cause premature deafness[61]. Try to reduce the amount of time you play music really loudly, especially if it is straight into your ears.

SUMMARY

- Eat a balanced diet.

- Take regular exercise.

- Limit your alcohol intake – see the chapter on addictions.

- Abstain from cigarettes and drugs – see the chapter on addictions.

- Eat nutrient rich food rather than taking supplements wherever possible.

- Get enough sleep.

- You need your body, so treat it well and be proactive about your health.

- Your body is part of you, not separate from you.

- Integrate all parts of yourself and work on physical, emotional, and mental health in a proactive manner.

- By taking these steps, you give yourself the greatest opportunity to live better and to keep going for longer!

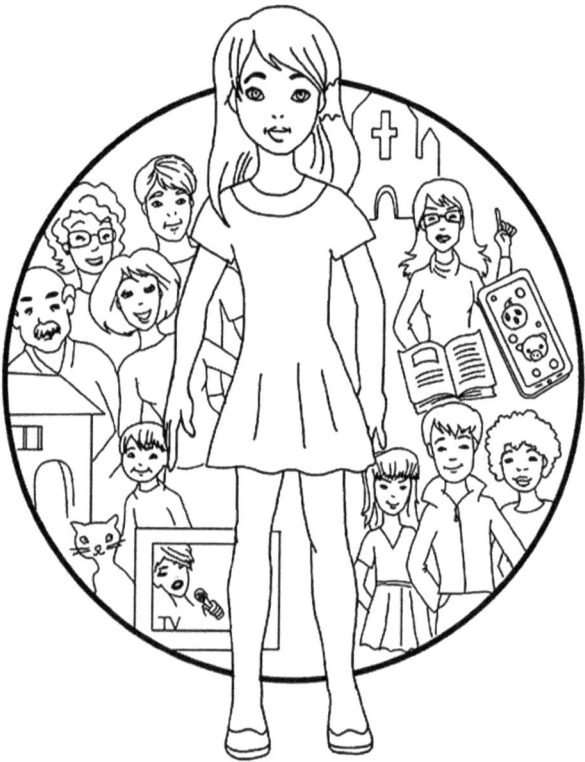

CHAPTER 3

FAMILY/HOME LIFE

*You can choose your friends,
but you can't choose your family.*

A family unit may consist of a variety of possibilities, and may comprise of a child or children being raised by a mother and father, a single parent, a blended family, a same sex couple, and so on.

The individuals may all live in one household, or may comprise people who live apart from one another, who can still be seen as the child or children's primary caretakers. The unit itself may change over time, and such changes may have consequences for a child's development.

THE IMPORTANCE OF FAMILY

The first seven to twelve years of life are very important in setting the tone for the rest of our lives. These are our years of growing up in all senses: physically, mentally and emotionally.

This is when the groundwork is laid down.

There is evidence that temperament is innate—or in your genes.

When babies are born, and in the early weeks and months, they can be categorised as warm or cold: this indicates whether or not a baby is particularly responsive to people and its surroundings.

It is debatable whether babies who are categorised as warm are necessarily what we might call extroverted when grown up. However, there could be at least a partial correlation.

In any case, 'warm' babies get more positive responses in a social sense than 'cold' babies who show very little response to others, so that as the baby grows where they are more responsive than more parental interaction occurs[62].

I would suggest that personality traits are a person's innate tendencies mixed with childhood experiences, where the innate tendencies may be a lot more detailed than just temperament.

There may be talents and interests that just need to be nurtured in the early years.

There appear to be a certain number of characteristics that are set at birth, but there are also a fair proportion that are due to the environment.

The current thinking on the nature/nurture debate appears to be that there is an integration of the two aspects in the expression of any particular characteristic, disease, or phenotype[63].

Very few genes control anything alone, and there are usually a number of genes implicated in any one thing. Genes may be either turned on or turned off, and environmental factors play a large role in effecting the outcome of your experiences.

This is why the early years are so important, and why having a loving and encouraging environment in a social sense is so important.

If an individual has a "good enough" early life this sets a good base to grow from.

A good enough upbringing means having overall positive experiences rather than negative experiences[64].

Negative experiences may override the positive ones—particularly if they are traumatic or complex.

Given that a baby is born with a nascent personality, then his or her personality is, to some extent, shaped by the experiences and incidences in his or her life as growth develops.

You may be born as an extrovert and also be adventurous. This will mean that you are into everything as a young child, and that you will approach others rather than holding back.

Such experiences will shape your resulting behaviour, if not your personality. Whether you get rebuffed or get approval for such behaviour will shape your *future* behaviour.

Where you have more positive experiences than negative, the good enough experiences come into play, and you will continue to approach others.

In this way, you are likely to make friends more easily, and so your personality grows.

NATURE/NURTURE

The issue of nature/nurture is still debated and researched.

Despite some things being set, there is still a lot of room to move. It seems that while about 45% is inherited, a great deal of how you behave in situations is up for grabs[65].

You can change your behaviour in many instances.

You may have been born with talents that you can practise to become good at.

If you are not assertive when young, then you can change and become more assertive. A pessimist may become more optimistic[66].

While some difficulties and disorders may not be totally resolved, there is certainly room for improvement from the baseline.

For example, anxiety may be inherited, but management may mean at least moderate relief[67].

POSSIBILITY

There is also the opportunity to discover things that will enhance your confidence, like practicing skills and behaviours, and finding the particular way to create the right environment within you and outside of you that will turn genes on or off. *You* are in charge of you, more so than your genes. You are in a dynamic interplay with your internal environment and your external environment, which gives you quite a bit of

---

> control if you decide to change your
> perceptions and interpretations of your world
> (in other words: change your mindset).

The environment of a child growing up is not only geological, but consists of the space of the immediate family, extended family, school, teachers, peers, media, church and religion, which all impinges on the curious and engaging mind of a child.

LEARNING AND MIRROR NEURONS

After birth, your brain is growing in size and the number of neurons and connections are increasing. Even before 12 months old, your capacity to copy and understand others is being developed. What really helps in this process is a kind of neuron called a mirror neuron. There are many of these mirror neurons in our brains, often forming clusters. These enable us to learn by association and to copy others' actions – firstly through observing what they are doing and being able to understand why they are doing that particular action[68]. This is where the mirror neurons come in.

When we watch someone carrying out a motor action – physical action such as grasping an object, our mirror neurons will be activated or firing as we watch. Then when we copy that same action, the same mirror neurons will again be firing exactly the same as when we were watching. What this means is that we are able to follow and understand the intent behind that action: thus, both the what and the why are understood.

There is evidence also that mirror neurons are involved in emotions and empathy. It appears that those people who are more empathic, through self-report in a questionnaire, tend to show stronger activations in their mirror neuron systems[69]

The mirror neuron system may also help us in our ability to develop our own theory of mind. This means that we can construct a model in our minds of the thoughts and intentions of others, and thus at least to some extent predict that person's behaviour[70]. This ability helps us to navigate the social environment within which we live.

The more experience you gain in life, and the more you know a particular person, the more clarity you will probably find in this ability. However, it does not mean that it is a perfect system. It just helps our brains make it easier to predict what may happen, and what is likely to keep us safe.

BELIEFS

As a child starts to make sense of his or her world, questions are asked.

Questions may be about things and animals, then later about why things are the way they are, how things work, and why—in this way, a picture is created.

In building a worldview, various beliefs are formed based on the explanations given from questions that are asked, and from interactions with the environment.

A belief is a statement about what we think happens in our world (both external and internal), and our worldview is built from the beliefs we form about what happens, how the world is, how other people are, and who we are, based on our experiences. Interactions with others and what we are told about ourselves are crucial in forming beliefs.

The more influence the person telling us about ourselves has on us, the more likely we are to believe it. However, the number of times we are told also affects how likely we are to take it on board.

Beliefs about ourselves are "core beliefs"[71].

There are considered to be ten core beliefs. They are: self-esteem, safety, competency, control, lovability, autonomy, justice, belonging, trust, and standards.

If you rate highly for all of these, or at least around the middle, then this is positive.

It will depend on your circumstances as to whether you rate low, medium or high for these core beliefs.

Sometimes, depending on recent past events, some core beliefs may become lowered for a time. However, it will be best if you can overcome such changes so that you can feel better about everything.

If you are interested in getting a rating of where you are in relation to these core beliefs, you can access a free survey at www.dianahutchison.com/shop.

Since only you will know your results, you can be honest. See what you get.

VALUES

Your parents and family are responsible for bringing you up, and this is where you get your ideas about yourself and the world, along with the later influences of preschool, day care, school and the children and adults you encounter along the way.

This is how your values and beliefs about you, your life, and the world are shaped. Your family is primary in you soaking up the values that are important to you in life. Values are the guiding principles of our life. It is helpful to sort out which values you feel are most important in your life.

You can download a free values survey at www.dianahutchison.com/shop. Rate each value out of ten, where ten is the most important. After you have rated each value, pick your top five.

Values differ across individuals and within individuals over time.

It is also helpful to think about how you incorporate these values into your life.

How do you express the importance of your values—how do you behave, what do you do? The expression of values varies across individuals.

For instance, for the value "achievement", one person may be motivated to do really well on tests and exams and achieve success in their career, while another may seek achievement in terms of their collection of memorabilia.

If you have worked out your top five values and figured out how you incorporate those values into your life, then you can start to think about how you view other people in relation to you, and in general. It is better to think well of others, particularly those you come into contact with and those close to you.

At the same time, it is important to be realistic, since we cannot get away from the fact that there are some pretty destructive people in the world.

INTERCONNECTEDNESS

Beliefs and the relationship with oneself impact on how values are incorporated into our lives.

If you believe that you are competent then you may value respect from others.

If you believe that others lie and cheat then you are not likely to show respect to them.

So, values, beliefs and, to some extent, attitudes to things are learnt in the home environment.

As a child becomes older a revision of beliefs and attitudes may occur. This is likely to happen after different beliefs and attitudes are encountered during a child's school years, and particularly when the child becomes a teenager.

This is a time when questions are asked and the teen places importance on peer relationships. If you negotiate this time in your life satisfactorily and manage to sort through all the contradictions and dichotomies presented to you, then you will maintain a sense of yourself as a good person.

HOME LIFE

Many young adults still live at home into their twenties and thirties.

It is usually cheaper and more convenient to do this, rather than living away from home. However, it is to be hoped that if you are doing this that you are making a reasonable contribution to expenses and chores in an adult fashion, rather than still living as a dependant.

When you are no longer a child you need to accept more adult responsibilities.

When you are earning an income, you could be contributing money towards rent, plus food money and something towards the cost of gas, electricity, and water.

You might want to work out a percentage that fairly represents your share.

If you are not able to pay as much as this, then maybe you have come to a mutual arrangement with your parent(s) to ensure you are contributing as much as you can and, ideally, also able to save money.

If you are in a share house or are living with a partner then you are likely to have more expenses. It all depends on your situation—whether you are working, living away from home, how many people you are living with, and their relationship to you.

In whatever situation you find yourself, it is important to divide up the expenses as evenly as possible. If you are living at home perhaps you can do your own laundry, including your bed linen, and vacuum your room on a regular basis, as well as the rest of the house from time to time, or you might clean the bathroom, sweep the yard, put out the garbage or any other chore.

Chores are part of life, and even though we might not relish having to do them, they help us get on with other activities and stop us living in squalor. While it might not be necessary to have an absolutely spotless house, it is preferable to have a generally clean house.

This is for health and hygiene reasons. It doesn't take much time to vacuum, do the dishes, mop down the floors and so on. You can do one thing at a time, and once it is done you don't need to do it again for a while. So, action rather than procrastination is called for.

If you are living at home you can negotiate with your parents regarding the chores you do that contribute to the household. You might cook a meal on a specific night or you might agree to do a couple of chores each week.

If you are in a share house then you might find it helpful to instigate house meetings and a roster for chores.

It depends on whether you share food or not, regarding which chores will be on the list. It might be good to put a certain agreed amount of money each week towards food and you could all go shopping together after you have made a shopping list.

Then you could have a roster for who does the cooking and who does the washing up. It would be helpful if the roster also included house-cleaning chores.

If you are living with your partner then you can have a discussion together and decide who is going to do what: however, this doesn't have to be a hard and fast rule. Divide up the chores so that the workload is 50/50, rather than one person doing less or more.

MOVING OUT OF HOME FOR THE FIRST TIME

When you are ready to move out of home you need to think about a number of things. For example, can you afford it?

To get a rental property, it helps to have a permanent job with a reasonable income. Budget for your move and save up. On top of the rent, you need the bond money, which is usually four weeks' rent.

Another question to answer is whether you are moving in with one or more friends or whether you will be living by yourself. This relates to how many bedrooms are needed in your rental property and how expensive it might be.

If you are moving in with friends, make sure to set up agreements around how you are going to share the expenses, whose name the utilities will be in, who will be taking up the lease, and whether the lease will be in one person's name or more.

Estimate utilities and budget for water, gas, and electricity per person, so you can all set aside enough money each week to cover these services.

You will probably need to supply yourselves with cutlery, crockery, pots and pans, bed linen, towels, as well as furniture. Work out who will contribute which items. Consider buying from op shops and second-hand shops, as this will save you a lot of money.

When looking for a rental property you need to put some time in.

It takes a bit of organisation to get to open inspections, have all the paperwork you need to put in an application for the property, and apply as soon as possible, if you are interested.

Watch out for gazumping—being outbid by other applicants.

If you have some good references and good employment then you may have an advantage over others. Good references make a big difference, so organise these in advance.

Applying online also seems to help, in order to not get left behind. However, even with all of this, it may take longer than you think to land yourselves a reasonable rental property.

At times, when the rental market is tight and there is not much supply, rents may rise and it may be difficult to afford a decent place to live. In these circumstances, renters are also likely to spend more of their income on housing, and therefore have less money available for daily living expenses and savings.

When you have secured a rental property then you need to organise yourself and your friends in order to take up occupancy. You will have a date from which the tenancy agreement begins, and you can move in after that, once you have the keys.

While you may be able to move quite a lot of stuff just using your car, some bigger items may need to be moved by a removalist company or with a truck or trailer, which you may be able to borrow or hire. Moving in is another expense that needs to be thought of in advance and allowed for.

BELONGING AND IDENTITY

Every human being wants to belong—to a family, a group, and a society. Human beings are social. We need each other to thrive.

It doesn't matter what racial background you have, you are part of many different groups, from the human race through to your family unit.

In multicultural societies and countries like Australia, the UK, Canada or the USA, it is becoming more important to accept everyone as part of your society.

No one is really different. Everyone has hopes and dreams, and each person should be respected as the unique individual they are.

All religious and political extremism that talks about hatred and violence towards others are to be avoided. These views are not humanistic nor helpful in adapting to human society as a whole.

Extremist views aside, in the global village we now have, we need to accept each other's differences. You don't have to agree with everything other people say or feel, but it is important to remember that there is more that unites us than divides us.

We are all the same underneath the skin, regardless of race, religion or colour.

Psychologically, we need to belong to a group. However, if we belong to a group then it follows that not everyone will necessarily belong to this group. Thus, there is an "in" group and an "out" group.

The "in" group will have characteristics that may be seen to be 'better' than those characterised by those considered to be the "out" group, and they may have privileges because of these characteristics.

The "in" group may then see themselves as better and may bully those who are not "in".

An experiment into this was first performed by Jane Elliot in 1968 in the USA[72].

Rules were given to an "out" group and "in" group, and privileges were given to the "in" group.

The teacher said that the kids with blue eyes were the "in" group.

Very quickly, the kids with blue eyes began to bully those with brown eyes.

The following day the teacher changed the rules and said that she had been mistaken, and those with brown eyes were actually better than those with blue eyes.

So, then the rules were reversed and all the kids in her class had the experience of being both part of the "in" group and the "out" group. Thus, every child in the class experienced how it felt to be part of each group.

The "blue eyes and brown eyes" experiment was an arbitrary grouping, but we group people arbitrarily all the time.

There may be any number of different ways in which people are grouped, although they are often based on ethnicity, race, colour, ability, gender, religion, and any other aspect that seems to create a distinction, and therefore a separation.

It is often just a matter of luck whether you belong to an "in" group or an "out" group.

Participants rarely have any say in the matter.

We should not blame those in the "out" group for being in the "out" group, or bully them for being themselves. Everyone belongs to the group of the human race. In reality, no one is "in" or "out". Every human being has equal rights to you.

FITTING IN/BELONGING

At school, fitting in is usually a case of finding friends to hang out with and working out where you are with your values and beliefs about yourself.

After you leave school, whether you go to work or higher education, this time is about working out where you fit in society. This may not necessarily be something you consciously seek, but it might nevertheless be a goal. If you can find something meaningful in your life then it might be your purpose.

Where you can find what you love doing this will help your life feel meaningful, whatever your interests are.

This is a time of working out what you believe in and also understanding how society functions. By degrees, it is possible to work out where you fit in, in context of the wider world of social interaction.

While there are varied beliefs and attitudes across society, not all are positive.

You will be on the right track if you search for beliefs that enhance the human spirit and do not endorse violence, hatred and revenge. If you look for beliefs that enhance the human spirit then you will find a more positive outlook, and increase your chances of a more optimistic and positive life that may include helping others.

As you go about your daily life you will find that society has norms and rules about how to interact with others. Because we are social beings, there are ways of behaving that tend to make it easier to relate to and deal with people.

One of these rules is manners.

It is polite to say please and thank you, and will more than likely get you what you want faster, or at least get a smile. When meeting new people, be interested in them. You may wish to ask them questions about themselves. By asking questions, you may find out something that will help you or a way in which you can help them. Small talk helps to grease the wheels of social interaction. Even just talking to others in a queue or talking to another briefly can give you a greater sense of connection. Depending on where you are meeting, it can lead to a deeper and more meaningful exchange and help you figure out if you have anything in common that might lead to a friendship.

It is important to talk inclusively and in a way that doesn't exclude various groups of people.

Society expects you to behave responsibly when you are an adult. This means behaving sensibly and within the law. If you can figure out where and how you fit in—even if only in theory—then feeling comfortable in society will be much easier.

WHEN THINGS GO WRONG
BREAKING THE LAW

If you break the law and it is a fairly minor crime, then you may only receive a caution or a fine. Getting into trouble with the police can feel very scary, and even a slight brush with the law may be enough to deter you from doing anything that will land you in trouble again.

If you find yourself in this situation then it can be a good opportunity to make changes to your life that ensure you stay out of trouble in future.

If you break the law while you are under eighteen years of age and it is serious, or if you have been in trouble many times before, then you might end up in juvenile detention.

Firstly, you'll be charged.

Secondly, you'll be locked up in a police cell until the next business day when you'll go to court to be granted bail. Whether bail is granted or not, you will be arraigned for a future date.

Arraignment is a formal reading of the charges being brought against you. It is at this stage that you may get a lawyer to represent you in court, either privately or through legal aid. However, legal aid lawyers are run off their feet with cases and may not be able to represent you in the way a private lawyer could.

In any event, you may need the evidence to be favourable in order to have the best outcome.

If you are granted bail then you are free to go back home, but you are obliged to attend court on the date that is set for your next hearing, and you may have bail conditions that place restrictions and demands on you which you must comply with in order to stay out of the remand centre. Bail conditions may include restrictions such as a curfew or no contact with any witnesses, and demands such as signing in at your local police station every day or every week, depending on how your risk level has been assessed.

Where bail is not granted then you will be taken to a remand centre for juveniles. In such an institution everyone is kept together, waiting to come to trial for their charges. You will probably need to share a cell with someone else.

You may or may not like them or get on with them. You may or may not get on with anyone there. There are likely to be power plays and even fights over seemingly inconsequential things.

Even small things in the outside world get to be important in custody.

In juvenile detention you are restricted in where you can go and what you can do, and you are constantly reminded that you have lost your freedom.

Visits only happen at certain times, such as weekends.

You are only able to purchase certain goods on buy-ups to take care of yourself and your habits.

You will have no access to a mobile phone.

If there are any computers, they will only be for use with educational courses, and not for personal use, and there will be no Internet access.

You will probably find that the officers are called "boss", or "chief", and that they have the say over everything while you are there. Roll call occurs at least twice a day.

A cast iron bladder is a positive.

While there are some programs that are available in detention, they are few and far between, so unless you want to do an educational course you will probably have little to do and be bored out of your brain.

In any case, while on remand the time frame for which you will need to stay there is uncertain, and could stretch from weeks to months or even possibly to years, so you will probably feel as though you are in limbo.

You will not like juvenile detention and it is not something to aspire to. No one will feel admiration for you going there and it is not something to big note yourself about.

ADULT JAIL

If you are eighteen years old or over when you commit a crime, then you will go into the adult prison system.

What holds for juvenile detention is doubly true for the adult system.

Both systems are hotbeds of crime.

You can learn more about how to commit various crimes, and come out as more of a hardened criminal rather than a reformed member of society. However, it is your choice and if you choose, you can make a jail sentence your call to a better life.

It is better if you make this call as a juvenile, but it will still work if you are in the adult system.

Take your sentence as a wake-up call and don't give in to the easy way. You have the opportunity to take your life into your own hands and make something of it. It is not too late. Get the support you need on your release and persevere.

There may be a number of reasons why young people, or even older people, get into crime and come to the attention of the police and the justice system.

A lot of the time, there are difficulties at home, and histories of trauma and violence, which then may lead to self-medication with alcohol and drugs, which then leads to more problems.

Sometimes it may begin with becoming part of a group or gang and getting a bit of an adrenaline rush through doing forbidden things, such as stealing cars and going for joyrides.

Whatever the reason, it is extremely important to understand that this type of behaviour is often a cry for help.

By healing the underlying issues in relation to the behaviour, whatever it is the result of, then behaviour change and deep inner change will occur. If this is you, then the best thing to do is to ask for help from the right people and organisations.

EXTREMISM

Extremism of any kind is often expressed by those on the margins of society. Staying within the central average block will still afford you a wide range of beliefs to choose from. Extremist beliefs are not enhancing to the human spirit and they do not help or enable people to live together in the world amicably.

How to recognise extremism:

- They have an exclusive "in" group that they invite you to join
- They make you feel special for joining
- They may have an initiation or ritual to join
- You get to belong to a select group with special privileges
- They preach hate, violence, vilification and discrimination towards those people in the "out" group
- They invite you to break laws
- They may require action on your part for accessibility for special treatment
- There may be money to be given to them, or some kind of imposition on you
- There could be long term negative consequences on your life and outcomes

Joining for social reasons and to belong somewhere doesn't work in the long run—there are alternative groups that will provide better, more positive emotions and a greater sense of belonging.

The Internet shows ranges of beliefs and attitudes, both politically and morally.

Sites espouse views from the far left of politics to the far right, including Neo-Nazi views. Anyone can set up a website and there are sites espousing what can be called "crackpot" views and conspiracy theories.

Be discerning and be careful. Sort out these websites, identify those indicating political extremes if you come across them, and don't pay attention to them.

A lot of websites cannot be trusted. It is better to pay attention to the websites that are more centrist and mainstream, especially if you are looking for balanced and accurate information.

Sites that talk about violence towards anyone and hold extreme views are not safe to explore, and it is dangerous to start to think like the people who create them and use them. Don't be swayed by what you read on these sites.

You would be best served by staying away from such views and maintaining a humanitarian stance.

POLITICS

It is also a time to work out where you stand in the political sense.

In Australia, where voting is compulsory, it is important to be aware of what you want to vote for. The issues that are important to you will be actioned if you vote for the party or people that have policies which address those issues. Become engaged and politically savvy.

Your vote, along with others of your generation, will make a difference. Read up and watch the political news, work out who you agree with, and vote for them when you have enrolled to vote.

One more recent place to find a balanced view of political news in Australia is 6News, which is sent out live on Facebook every weekday night.

This is a channel run by teenagers, who are growing up fast.

The first step you need to take in order to vote is to enrol when you turn eighteen years old. If you haven't enrolled yet and you are older, then do it now.

Work out where you stand on the party policies of each party, and vote accordingly. Some issues may be more important to you and so you might concentrate on your most important issues. It shouldn't just be about your own benefits, but rather the benefits of the many and of your country. Social justice should figure in your thoughts. In other words, think of others and the larger picture, rather than just yourself.

INTERPERSONAL BEHAVIOUR

Some people work hard to do the right thing by others.

It is important to treat others the way *you* would like to be treated. It is not enough to treat others how they treat you. This is more likely to get you into a downward spiral of assuming something, acting on it, and not getting the results you were after in the first place. If you always *treat others how you would like to be treated* then this means that others will have a positive view of you and will therefore be happy with you, and you will be more likely to get the results that you want.

It is, however, not just getting the best for yourself – if you always treat others how you would like to be treated then you are acting from a good humanitarian value base.

SUMMARY

- Move towards humanitarian values and the humane, rather than the extremes.

- Become aware of the whole world rather than just your world.

- Become interested in politics and the environment, and act on a local level. You may even inspire others.

- Think about social justice and follow your heart.

- Keep family relationships as positive as you can.

- By taking these steps you can create a peaceful family or home life.

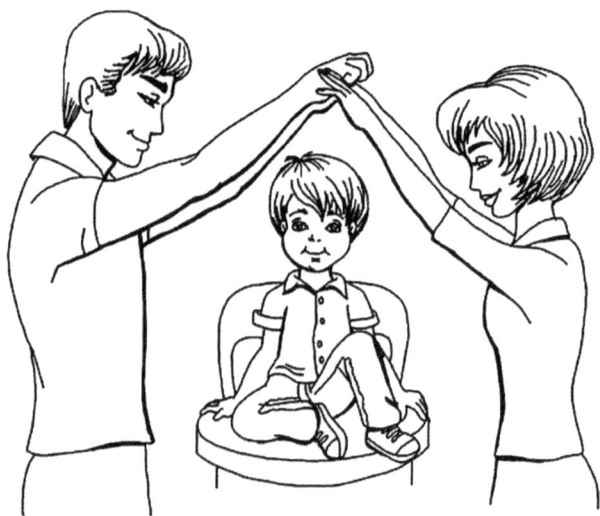

CHAPTER 4

RELATIONSHIPS

What kinds of relationships bring you joy?

The relationships we have with others help to connect us.

When we feel connected, we thrive. The quality of our relationships affects how we feel about ourselves and our lives. Relationships affect us on all levels: physically, mentally, emotionally, and spiritually.

The social support you have helps you through troubled times and allows you to be happier and healthier than otherwise.

Having four to five close friends makes for a happier and less lonely person[73],[74]. Additionally, those with partners or who are married generally have a better quality of life than those who are single [75]. However, it is the case that if your situation is contrary to how you actually want it, then you may be less happy and thus not have as great quality of life.

What this means is that those who do not want

children or to necessarily marry are happier later in life because this was their choice[76].

It makes sense to work on your relationships because they are so important. Become the best friend and the best partner you can be. As you change and grow within yourself, your relationships will also change and evolve.

The best relationship may occur when each person is accepted and respected for themselves and the relationship together continually evolves.

FAMILY

It is important for a baby to feel cared for so that his or her needs are met.

If their needs are met most of the time, then this is 'good enough' parenting and the baby will have an overall positive experience.

Security is essential for a baby and for a child.

When a child is a bit older, it is important to set boundaries, so then the child will be secure in knowing the limits of behaviour. This will mean that later on he or she can be a well-functioning member of society, and will be able to set their own limits.

While Bowlby[77] first brought the idea of "good enough" mothering into use and discussed attachment theory, Dan Hughes[78] is a more recent attachment theorist.

A baby attaches to his or her attachment figures for comfort and safety—including for food, warmth, and protection.

The baby interacts with the attachment figures with eye contact, nonverbal communication and touch. The response a baby receives from his or her caregivers determines whether he or she becomes securely or insecurely attached. Responses can range from consistently welcoming and warm to distant and irregular. Again, if the response is positive, then the baby will become securely attached. If generally the response is negative, then the baby will develop an insecure attachment.

Through our attachment histories we tend to utilise generally consistent approaches to our relationships over time. Thus, patterns of thought, emotion, and behaviour may be noticed over relationships, and between them too.

A secure attachment in childhood means that you are more likely to become an independent and autonomous adult. In this case, healthy relationships will eventually form. This is more likely because in a secure attachment, a child is able to learn more about themselves and about the world, since they feel safe to explore it. If you had a healthy, secure attachment as a child you would have felt safe with your caregiver and been able to feel safe in novel situations and thus more brave in exploring your environment around you.

In an insecure attachment, a child learns much less about themselves and the world, and learns less from his or her parents at the same time[79]. Insecure attachment can mean challenges in forming healthy relationships in your life.

Whatever your attachment pattern, it is possible to become more autonomous and independent as an adult and display more attributes of a secure attachment style.

As an adult our attachments styles may be:

1. **Preoccupied** - where a person is continually preoccupied with the relationship to the detriment of the relationship itself;

2. **Dismissive** - where a person is dismissive of the relationship and minimises the extent of it and issues around it;

3. **Unresolved** - where there is no coherent pattern and relationships are problematic

4. **Autonomous** - where a secure attachment was formed as a baby. The person is independent and confident in relationships.

Family relationships are very important. If you received good enough parenting as a baby and child then you are likely to be secure in yourself, since your family relationships were stable and secure.

Quarrelling with siblings is normal, provided it's not all the time.

Where family life was unstable for any reason as a young child, then you are more likely to feel less secure and you may not feel as good about yourself as you otherwise would.

ATTENTION!

If you are currently experiencing or have recently experienced family or relationship problems that are affecting you and upsetting you a great deal, it may be a good time to find someone who might be able to listen to you and help you understand and sort out how to manage your situation. Where you feel you cannot approach family members, then a person outside of the family may be best. You could try helplines (such as Headspace and Kids Helpline in Australia) for a start. It is much better to be proactive and ask for help when you need it rather than staying stuck and not knowing the best ways to think, feel or act.

Where you had more negative than positive experiences, had a dysfunctional family, or experienced traumatic events, all is not lost.

Children are resilient, and from the vantage point of an adult, many of these issues may be worked upon and the effects lessened to a reasonable extent, and any effects may or may not occur in the first instance[80]. Asking for help from a trained professional would be a recommended action.

You are not defined by those experiences that have not been helpful. There are relationships beyond the family that may be of more positive use.

You can choose to use these as your positive point of reference.

Negative feelings from relationship experiences are normal and are part of recognising what an unhealthy relationship is. This is how you can use your negative experiences in a positive way.

BOUNDARIES

Boundaries are the limits we set on acceptable behaviour. Boundaries should be put in place early so that a child is able to feel secure and safe.

Parents can still be loving and set boundaries. When boundaries are set a child will be able to take responsibility for his or her actions, attitudes, and emotions, based on his or her experience.

There are good boundaries and unhealthy boundaries. How do you recognise them?[81] Everyone needs to have personal boundaries. These are limits on yourself and others, in relation to behaviour. To have healthy boundaries in place means that you are able to be assertive and relate your limits to others in a way that takes their needs into account, as well as your own needs.

In a family, the parents have a boundary around them[82]. They share confidences and intimacy that they do not share with their children. They share more information with their children, but it is different—they should not share personal information and confidences with their child that would normally be shared with a partner. If they do, then enmeshment occurs and the boundary that should exist between parent and child is breached. Enmeshment is a condition in which two or more people, typically family members, are involved in each other's activities and personal relationships to an excessive degree, thus limiting or stopping healthy interaction and compromising individual autonomy and identity[83]. Children do not know how to deal with adult confidences and should not be asked to do so. Children should also not be placed in a situation where they need to act as a go-between or to choose between the parents. This is another form of enmeshment[84].

When it comes to personal boundaries, there are areas in which it may be helpful to consider where your boundaries are in relation to others. Sharing information with others requires clarity in how much you are prepared to share with whom. You are probably likely to share more personal information with family and those you are close to, than those you don't know as well, or who are strangers. In addition, there are the different areas in which you may have boundaries.

These include physical, intellectual, emotional, sexual, material, and time boundaries. For a time boundary, for example, if you have not thought about this or defined what your wishes are in this respect, then you may find yourself allowing others to take up your time, even in a situation where you wanted to do something instead. Even if you find yourself giving someone more time than you would want one time, you can always get clear on your wishes, and put a clearer boundary into place next time.

It is said that boundaries may be porous, or firm (ideal). The clearer you can be on your boundaries (and what you share) and where you stand in relation to what you will accept from others, the easier it will be to navigate relationships in general.

No matter what your boundaries, see *Ten Ways to Build and Preserve Better Boundaries*[85]. There are some good tips you can put into action now.

HOW TO SET BOUNDARIES

In order to navigate life and to relate with others in a meaningful way, we need to understand where we stand—with ourselves and others. Consciously deciding on our boundaries is essentially the best way to move forward in relationships. Sticking to your boundaries, while they continue to be relevant, will serve you best.

Boundaries in relationships describe how much you share with others, particularly personal information, and how much detail you provide. Having healthy boundaries is based on equality, mutual respect, and honesty. Treating others respectfully is a great basis for positive relationships.

If you have already decided on how much personal information you are going to share with friends, and which particular friends you share things with, and what it is you are willing to share with them, and what you are not willing to do with them, you will hold the key to opening the door to better communication in your relationships.

You don't necessarily need to proclaim your boundaries unless you realise others are crossing those boundaries you have set for yourself.

You can set boundaries and limits for yourself and for others. This means healthy boundaries that help you feel safer, more together, whole, and clear— not unhealthy restrictions or demands that you use to control other people. Setting healthy boundaries will not only help you, but will also allow the other person to feel you are respecting them as a person who can take responsibility for themselves.

When a boundary is crossed by another, then it is important to immediately speak up. Say what your boundary is, in terms of behaviour and the limit being placed upon the person. In addition, you can say what the consequences will be for breaking the boundary again. It is helpful to have perhaps three different consequences going from the first time to the third time, with increasingly hard consequences.

For instance, a boundary might be that people should listen to what you are saying, without interrupting.

The first-time infraction might get a warning of what will occur if there is a second time.

The second time, perhaps the consequence is that the person loses a minor privilege. The third time, the person might lose something more important.

The boundary needs to be set verbally with the person concerned and the consequences spelt out before you start counting infringements. For information on how to set boundaries for children see[86].

You can also set a boundary for yourself. You may enjoy going to the pub with your friends, but you may also need to get up early for work during the week. You might set a boundary so that you stay at home and go to bed early during the week, and only go to the pub on Friday and Saturday nights.

This boundary means you sometimes miss out on something that you enjoy, in order to ensure you can get up for work on time and have a clear head. By ensuring you are able to perform well at work, you also ensure you can continue to fund your social life and enjoy your weekends out with your friends. In this way, setting a boundary means that both your professional and your social life are sustainable in the longer term, even if you are making some sacrifices in the short term.

When setting boundaries for yourself and for others, you need to ensure that you stick to your rules, and carry out the consequences when appropriate.

It may be easier to set boundaries for others and stick to them than sticking to boundaries that you set for yourself. It does take practice to stick to your own boundaries. However, even if you forget or ignore a boundary you have set for yourself once, then it is still possible to put it in place next time.

It may take a bit of effort but it could well be worthwhile continuing to work at enforcing your boundaries. Setting boundaries for yourself may well be very similar to putting new routines into your life and changing your behaviour.

See my first book for tips on how to create positive and sustainable change. www.amazon.com/author/dianahutchison

ROLE MODELS

The family is a blue print for how we relate to others in the world.

Our primary caretakers model the behaviour, and we view this behaviour as the way to do things in relationships.

Your primary caretakers are your first role models.

This relates to both the behaviour seen between them as well as how they behave towards you, your siblings, and others outside of the family. As you grow up and have your own family, you might catch yourself behaving like your parental figures. While you may take this behaviour as a model for your behaviour, it is also possible that you take their behaviour as a model for how *not* to behave. It could go either way.

The process of using their behaviour as a model works quite well where you have had good enough parenting yourself, but can fall over where you haven't. In this circumstance, it is helpful to have a positive role model within your wider circle of extended family, friends, or community members.

Although our parents are our first role models, we may choose other role models when we are a little older. These are people we admire and want to be like.

Such role models may be known to you through school, family connections or friends. It is helpful if you choose your role models carefully.

As we grow up, where we are heterosexual and grow up in a similar two-parent family, we probably use the same sex parent as a role model, and use the opposite sex parent as an aspiration for an intimate relationship.

If you are female then you may find yourself attracted to men who are like your father in some way. If you think about it, there may be an issue that is repeated in your relationships with men your own age that was an issue between you and your father.

Similarly, with men and their mothers. If you are homosexual then the issue may be similar to the same sex parent, but it might not.

The issue may not necessarily be a problem, but it might indicate such things as characteristics you are attracted to.

However, there may be an underlying problem depending on the parent's behaviour. Psychologically, we are attracted to those people who will present us with the issues we need to resolve (this being a conditioning aspect in our brains which no longer serves us). So, if your father left the family home or died when you were young, then you may find yourself attracted to men who tend to abandon you. If this is the case then you could face the issue straight on and have counselling to resolve it.

Once you resolve these issues you will be able to change the quality of partner you end up with.

Similarly, if a man's relationship with his mother has been very intense then he may continue to have difficulties with partners. If there are issues, they will always be specific to the individuals involved. It is a good idea to look underneath the surface interactions in your relationships so that you can be aware of the undercurrents and the motives you have, as well as those that your partner has.

Your parents are likely to have your best interests in mind. Understand this when they warn you off from being with certain people and from doing certain things.

Be willing to discuss all aspects and reasons why they think this way.

The more they are willing to talk about it and explain their reasons, your understanding improves, and you will be empowered to make the decision that is right for you.

As we grow up, we interact with our family members. Your ways of talking, in terms of what you say, how you say it, when, and why you say it, will depend on your family interaction experience. Were you continually put down for saying things or were you encouraged to speak your mind?

Whatever pattern occurred in your family will have

an effect on how you now communicate.

Did your parents model good communication styles such as assertiveness?

Was each family member given the space and respect to say their piece?

There will be some effect of such practices on your ability and willingness to communicate with others—even if there is only a small effect, there will still be an effect.

If you are a tween or a teenager, then these times may be somewhat difficult on a few fronts.

Firstly, biologically, hormones are starting to kick in and your body may be starting to change, or has already. This means that your circadian rhythms may also have changed. It is now known that the circadian rhythms of teenagers up to early adulthood shift, so that their sleeping patterns move to later times.

This means that they stay awake later and cannot get going until later in the morning. This is why it is difficult to get out of bed early.

If this is you, then it is not your fault[87].

Unfortunately, school does not cater for this and being tired does not help the learning process.

Other factors in play for teenagers include a greater pull to peer relationships, and sometimes (but not always) a differentiation from parental values and ideas. This may be difficult or not, but it is certainly a time when you are becoming more your own person and coming to realise you can create your own life. In this exploration, it can be helpful to be discerning and cautious around those people you associate with and whom you feel you want to be like.

SCHOOLING PLUS

There will also be an effect on your relationships based on your experiences at school, and your personality may have impacted your school relationships.

Things such as whether you make friends easily or not, whether you become popular or not, and whether you are bullied or not. Possibly, your respect for your parents will relate to the respect you have for your teachers.

Your school experiences may affect

- your idea of yourself as an agent of action and change

- how you see yourself as a person
- your beliefs about yourself and the world
- self-esteem, competence, and other core beliefs

There is no excuse for bullying, just as there is no excuse for physical violence. Verbal violence is also very damaging and shows difficulties with learning how to relate to people in a respectful and meaningful way.

Bullies may learn by their parents modelling the behaviour, or they may be essentially insecure and see their bullying as a way of making themselves more secure in their relationships with their friends. School is a place where any difference may be noticed and attacked, whether by teasing or bullying. In any case, bullying is not a nice thing to engage in and puts the victim into a negative emotional state.

While it is the case that most schools have anti-bullying programs in place, bullying still may occur whether in person or online, and this may have dire consequences in some instances.

Dealing with verbal bullying can be really tough. Sometimes, it's hard not to let the hurtful words get to you, but remember, they're just someone else's opinions, not facts about who you are. Believing in yourself and your strengths is crucial. Don't let the bully's words define you. It certainly hurts but remember that you have control over how you respond to it. By talking about it with the right people, you can find ways to cope with the emotional and psychological impact. You don't have to face this alone; there are people who care about you and want to help. It's totally okay to reach out to someone you trust, like a teacher, employer, family member, or friend, and talk about what's going on. They'll be there to support you and help you come up with ways to handle the situation.

One way to manage it is to use creative visualisation: using your imagination, see the following image in your mind.

Imagine you have a strong stone wall around you, as high as you want it and that anything that is hurtful bounces off the wall and returns back to the speaker.

You can in fact create whatever will work for you. If you think a different image will work better, then use that. You might put yourself into a metal sphere, or any other kind of structure that words will bounce off and return to the sender.

This is just one way to deal with it. It will depend on the situation and whatever your circumstance is, exploring options for support and strategies that may work for you will be a positive option.

When physical bullying occurs, it often coincides with other forms of bullying, predominantly psychological in nature. It encompasses inappropriate touching, acts of violence, or any behaviour that causes you to feel discomfort. These actions invade personal boundaries, and encroach upon one's personal space. When physical harm is inflicted, it constitutes a clear violation. However, other forms of bullying are equally detrimental. Any type of bullying, whether physical or psychological, can inflict lasting psychological damage. The ultimate consequence of bullying is the erosion of one's sense of safety, along with self-confidence and feelings of self-worth. Bullying can be insidious, and its impact may be felt even if the victim remains silent due to discomfort.

FRIENDSHIPS

We usually become friends with people with whom we have something in common. We stay friends if the common interaction grows into liking and the relationship helps to fulfil our needs of friendship and association.

Someone is an acquaintance if they are not well known but you spend some time with them on occasions.

With a friend, you can share quite a lot about yourself and they will share themselves too, so that you end up with quite a strong bond.

The more time you spend together and the more you share yourself then the more likely it is you have a strong friendship.

Of course, it does depend on the personalities of those involved, and that needs to be taken into account in any analysis of the friendship. It is helpful to at least occasionally look at motives and intent for behaviours you observe.

In this way you will know them better and you can come to a conclusion, in some form, about your friendship.

By observing behaviour, it is possible to infer motive and, additionally, you have the luxury of being able to ask your friend what motivated him/her. From this conversation you will come to know your friend better. There can be different expectations from friendships between girls and boys, and these expectations can increase during adolescence[88].

To be a good friend, it is important to encourage the other person to achieve their goals, to support them on the way and to lend a sympathetic ear.

You don't need to fix their problems. You just need to listen. By all means make a suggestion, but it is your friend's life and only they are responsible for their own life. You can strongly advise your friend to do or not to do something that is in their long-term interest, but if they still decide on a certain action then you can't change that.

It is helpful to look at long-term consequences when making decisions to act in a certain way. Although this is not the first and easiest way of thinking when one is a young adult, it will serve you well if you start putting it into practice.

Ask yourself, 'If I do act, then what are the long-term consequences?'

For example, if it involves drinking alcohol then you need to bring into account the effects of binge drinking on your behaviour, your brain, and your memory.

Then you can ask yourself, 'Does this particular behaviour help me fulfil my values?' After that, you can think about the short and medium-term consequences, such as having fun with your friends. You can also advise your friends to make their decisions based along these lines. Whatever decisions they ultimately make will be up to them.

The same process can be taken when you feel that you are under pressure to engage in behaviour that might be risky or have negative consequences. Peer pressure can be a very strong force when we are young, because we need to feel that we belong— and in order to belong we think that we need to 'join in' with others. This idea, to some degree, is in our heads. Friends are not necessarily going to drop you just because you don't go along with them on occasion, or engage in a particular behaviour. If they do, then you are probably better off without them, and if they don't drop you then you know they are true friends.

The important aspect to this is that you are true to yourself and don't get swept up into being someone you don't want to be or doing things you don't want to do.

The issue is that these things need to be thought of and decided on *before* the situation arises, because peer pressure and the heat of the moment can lead you in the wrong direction.

If you have made a firm decision prior to the occasion and have worked out what you will do (setting boundaries), then when the occasion arises you will be able to recognise it and take action— whether this means that you leave the situation or try to convince your friends against it. You will know that you have done the right thing by yourself and others, including society.

The question of legalities should also be taken into account when making decisions, not just risk and possible consequences. If it's illegal, the safest option is not to do it, because the consequences might be catastrophic. It is not enough to believe that you are bulletproof, that you won't get caught or that nothing bad will happen; you *aren't* bulletproof, you may well get caught, and that bad things do happen. The more you act within the law, the less likely it is that negative consequences will occur.

Laws are made for the wellbeing of society. If you don't drink and drive, don't use drugs, and don't drive above the speed limit then you are less likely to have a road traffic accident, and, therefore, less likely to die or be incapacitated for the rest of your life. More incidents of death and incapacitation occur for young males between sixteen and twenty-four than any other group. You could start a habit of thinking about the possible consequences of your behaviour. This could help you avoid situations you might otherwise find yourself in.

One way to think about your safety is that your body is your temple—it is yours alone. You are in charge of it and have the right to say what you do with it.

Because you are on a lifelong journey with it, you need to be aware of the consequences of actions and practices that may have a detrimental effect on your physical body, your psychology, and your sense of self.

Sometimes, your safety physically can be fine, but your psychological state and sense of self may be compromised through those that you may associate with. If you are in a group of people that you find appear to either reject you or put you down in some way so that you end up feeling any of the following, then this may be an unhealthy friendship group for you.

If you feel that:

- you are being taken advantage of
- you are being used
- your values are being over-ridden by what you are doing
- you just don't want to be a part of what you are doing then you need to take a step back.

If you find yourself in this situation, the best thing you can do is say, 'No' to going out with your friends. Despite the fact that you will feel pressured into going out and doing the things they want to do, it is good in this instance to be strong and not go. The point might be that they are not really your friends, and you may be able to find a better group of friends that will not use and abuse you, or act in ways that are illegal or immoral. It may be tough to say no, but you need to put yourself first.

CLOSE RELATIONSHIPS

Being in a close relationship does not mean that you can't have friends and hobbies outside of that relationship. In fact, it is a good idea to have at least a few things that the two of you don't share.

It is better for mental health and overall wellbeing. Then when you do come together for those things you share you will be able to be enthusiastic about them.

In any relationship, communication is the key to success. That means communication both ways. It is best to be honest and up front about everything. While you might share some things about yourself with your friends, you might share everything with your partner, so that they may know you and trust you more.

If something happens and that trust is lost then it takes quite a long time to get that trust back again. At the same time, you may keep a few things to yourself.

Essentially, it's quite ok to keep a few things to yourself. Obviously, talking about the minute details of how you think about particular subjects is not obligatory.

There are boundaries to set around the amount of sharing that takes place, as well as time spent together, and financial boundaries too in relation to how much you share together and what limits you put on this. The biggest boundary is in relation to behaviour—discuss what you like, dislike and want in a close relationship.

Equality, respect, and consent are most important.

Read further for more on consent. For more tips on building healthy relationships see[89].

It is helpful to communicate assertively, so that both partners know where they stand, can ask for what they want within the relationship, and get their needs met. Sometimes it's the case that one partner may be dominant and the other more submissive. This is not always positive for the more submissive partner.

It depends on the personalities involved and the behaviours that are involved, as well. The more equal each partner can be in the relationship, the better.

If you are able to talk and communicate your thoughts, feelings, and ideas to your partner, and vice versa, then you have a good basis for a relationship.

Every now and then it is a good idea to sit down and discuss how you both see the relationship, and where you see it going.

Are you both getting your needs met? Are you both happy? Would you like something to change? Would you like to do more things together, or would you like more time for your own pursuits?

The more honest and open you are the better you will be able to communicate.

One difference between males and females seems to be that males are not always comfortable talking about emotions and feelings, whereas many females like doing this.

If you are male, particularly if you are in a heterosexual relationship, and you like to fix things, then learn to be ok with listening to your partner talk about her feelings without trying to provide solutions. You don't need to fix anything—by listening and responding in the right way you will be helping your partner to feel better.

Active listening is a key factor in this process.

What active listening involves is repeating some of the other person's words back to them in a way that affirms their experience. For example, if your partner says they are upset about something, say to them 'you feel upset'. This will indicate to them that you are listening and understand what they are feeling. They will then be able to say more about the situation. They will feel that they are heard. Whether you are in a heterosexual or a same sex relationship, whether you are a man who is comfortable talking about his emotions with a male or female partner who finds it difficult to discuss feelings, or whether neither partner finds emotional conversations easy, these ways of understanding the other person may be helpful. It doesn't matter who the person is who wants to fix stuff, that person needs to pay attention to active listening and help their partner in this process. If each of you is able to actively listen to the other then communication will be good.

ACTIVE LISTENING EXERCISE

A. Work is no good right now. Every time I try to do something right, I get criticised. It really upsets me.

B. You feel upset when you get criticised

A. Yes, and I'm not sure how to do things differently so that I don't get criticised.

B. You're unsure what to do.

A. Yes. What might be best?

B. What are your options as you see them?

In this conversation B is helping A to move forward and process her feelings. A gets to the point of problem solving in a short time as she feels heard and understood.

CONSTRUCTIVE EXERCISES

An exercise that you can do is to count the negative to positive statements that you say to your family members or partner, and their statements to you.

This ratio is called the Losada Ratio and it is an important indicator of the health of the relationship.

If it is 3:1 (negative to positive) then you are in trouble. If it's 1:2.9 you are ok, but if it's 1:5 then your relationship is terrific. In counting this ratio, it is best to use single sentences and take turns in speaking. See[90] for a more in-depth look at this.

One goal that comes out of this, however, is that if you are interested in improving your relationships you need to increase the number of positive statements you use. This may take some time to manage, but if you go through the process of setting the goal, monitoring your behaviour and putting new behaviours in place as discussed in my previous book, *A Practical Guide for Self Change*[91], then you will be well on your way.

If you have some constructive criticism to give someone, then the best way to do this is in a sandwich of positive statements. For instance, you could say, 'I love the meals you make when it's your turn to cook. It would be great if you could give the kitchen a bit of a clean as you go along, to keep everything organised, in the same way you organised the brilliant system of writing on the kitchen blackboard when we're running out of something.'

This sandwich helps the other person to be buoyed up by the positive statements, and although he or she will hear the criticism they are more likely to take it on board because of the way it has been delivered.

MANAGING EXPECTATIONS

In any close relationship, sex is an important component. Consent is crucial in any sexual encounter.

Communication is a key issue here. Negotiating intimate relationships can be difficult, but it can be done. Look at co-dependence and dependency. Make sure that you are not making the other person responsible for *your* responsibilities. Look at whether you need the other person to be a certain way.

If, for instance, a number of your partners have had addiction issues, then you may be co-dependent and trying to rescue them. It is impossible to change other people—they have to do it themselves. Instead, change your own patterns and find a partner who is different.

Nowadays, there is online dating.

Expectations here also need to be managed. When you meet people online you may gain an initial perception of them. Communications online can become quite intense. However, this may just be online, and the reality when you meet them may be very different.

So, you need to keep your feet on the ground and try not to build your expectations up too much.

One thing about online dating is that when you do meet them, you may know a bit more about them than most people you meet face-to-face for the first time. It is also worth keeping in mind that people may not be who they say they are.

At the very least, this could lead to disappointment. At the very worst, you could put yourself in danger from scammers or people with violent tendencies.

When meeting someone in person that you have met online, whether through a dating app, social media platform or otherwise, always tell someone where you are going and make sure you meet in a public place.

Since there are more dating apps available now, and since meeting strangers does not always lead to great experiences, it is important to protect yourself from having your drink spiked or other nasty actions. Sometimes there is safety in numbers, but not always.

Have safeguards in place where possible.

GENERALLY SPEAKING

It's important that you feel in control of yourself. It's even better if you feel in control of your life. You need to feel that you are in charge of yourself and therefore have an equal part in forming effective relationships.

If you are always doing what others want then think about what this means for your own behaviour and identity. Perhaps it is ok if you sincerely want to do what others want you to do, but if there are times when you only go along with others because you feel you can't say no then please see the chapter on assertiveness and meeting your needs.

Do you make suggestions about outings, and are they considered?

Do you feel that others notice you, care about you and are willing to go along with you?

The answers to these questions will show you where you feel you have agency and where improvements could be made. Even though it might not feel like it, one area where you do have agency is in the ways you can change yourself, if you so desire.

You can change yourself, but you can't change others. If you change first then others may change their behaviours towards you. Whether or not they do, it is a good idea to focus on self-change.

At times, throughout our relationships, revealing our vulnerable side is a good idea. Showing vulnerability helps others to understand us better and to trust us more. It also means that we become stronger within ourselves and more confident in who we are.

Being vulnerable sometimes shows others, especially our partner, that we trust them. It is most helpful in a heart-to-heart discussion about the relationship. It can help a relationship to grow, and can be used at various times to reveal little known information or secrets about oneself that may be shared in a close relationship.

FROM TEEN TO ADULT

Once you transition from being a teen to a young adult, the expectation of society is that you now have responsibility for your own behaviour. Behaviour may lead to consequences, and you need to accept this.

Society also expects that you will become a contributing member. So it is at this time, when turning eighteen years old, that you can start to think about behaviour and consequences more than in the past.

Many cultures have a rite of passage that marks the transition from childhood to adulthood as its focus. Eighteenth birthday parties, and various other events to mark specific ages or transitions are included here.

The way you transition to being an adult is very individual. If you have accepted the idea of responsibility then you are more likely to take yourself and your world a little more seriously than others who have not. It helps to have discussions around what happens in the world, particularly around behaviour and possible consequences.

It is, however, the application of this idea to oneself that is important.

Some people do not get it, and others get it, but carry on regardless.

It is possible to engage in taking on responsibility in a gradually increasing way. Thus, if you are in higher education, you can take on responsibility for your own learning.

To achieve this, you would be doing more study, completing the readings, doing the suggested extras and making sure that your assignments are in on time.

Where you find work, then you can accept responsibility for your performance, and can make sure that you are a model employee. Where you can't find work then you can still take responsibility for your search.

You can send in applications, ensure they are the best you can make them, do your best at interviews, and generally try hard to find work.

At the same time as you are engaging in these behaviours and taking responsibility for yourself, there is also your social life to consider. Just as with your education and employment, the more responsibility you can apply here, the better.

The older you get, the easier it is to see the connection between behaviour and consequences. When you do become more responsible and consider others as well as yourself, then you become a true adult. This acceptance may come earlier or later, depending on you.

SELF-ASSESSMENT

You could carry out a survey of your family and

friends and ask them how they would describe you as a person.

Write down their responses—don't judge them, but see them as a starting point to a better you. What you are getting is baseline data about how you come across to others. You could also ask your family and friends the questions, 'What do you think would help me to become better?' and, 'How do you think I could change?'

If those you ask are answering honestly and sincerely, you should get a result that provides some indication of future goals that you could action and achieve, should you so decide.

You then have the choice of working out how you want to be as a person and what identity you project. There are some things that are very difficult to change about ourselves, but it is possible to become better at things such as being assertive, and getting on with people.

Additionally, you can improve your skills, and learn new things. As you do these things you also may change your beliefs, values, ideas and attitudes.

SUMMARY

- Take responsibility for yourself, at home, school or work, and in your social life.

- Keep your activities legal.

- Make sure that you are treating your body with respect and say no when you want to.

- Be open and honest in your relationships.

- Ask your friends for feedback so you can get some ideas about what you can do to improve yourself and your relationships.

- By taking these steps, your relationships can start becoming awesome.

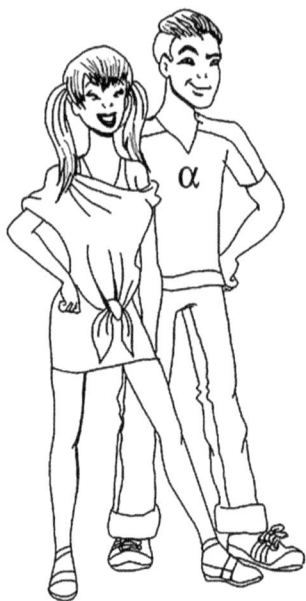

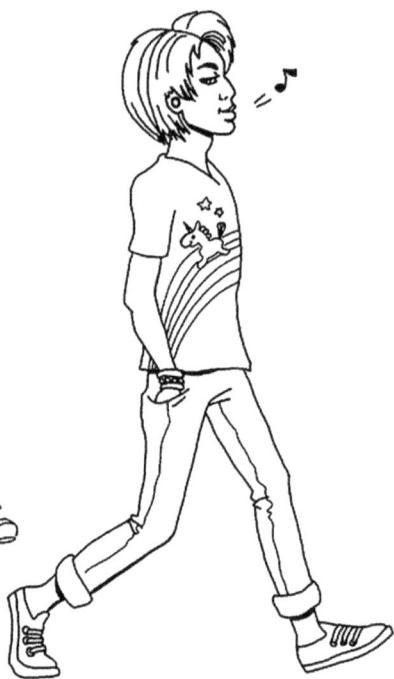

CHAPTER 5

SEX AND SEXUALITY

How do you identify as a sexual being?

Sexual identity and sexual orientation are innate, this means you are born that way. Neither sexual identity nor sexual orientation is open to change[92]. You feel you are a male or female, and you are attracted to males or females—or both. Sexuality and gender are both being increasingly recognised as a spectrum. Everything is ok no matter who you are; discovering and accepting yourself, no matter what, is important. Nature produces a mix of sexual identities and orientations, and we need to see all these differences as natural, because they are.

Where there are differences that an individual can change to enhance his or her life, then this change is appropriate.

Sexual preferences are laid down in late childhood, up to the time when puberty kicks in. Preferences revolve around orientation, you might like bums, breasts, and so on. When the preference focuses on usual aspects, then that is considered "normal". When the preference is unusual, such as some kind of object such as shoes, for example, then it is called a fetish. Once formed, preferences endure[93].

COMING OUT

Children easily identify what is accepted as "normal" in society. Because the predominant story is straight and heterosexual, difference is not always accepted by everyone. It is usual for those children who do not fit into the "norm" to feel that they are different when quite young.

Consciously identifying where you fit in may not always occur as a teen, but because sexual identity is now becoming more fluid for young people, and is becoming more accepted in many societies, then hopefully timelier "coming out's" may occur.

Working out your sexual identity, from childhood up, can be a time of inner turmoil and conflict. There may be bullying and problems at school. The Internet is not far away, and you can find "coming out" stories online, so that you will not feel so isolated.

Since this time is so confusing and full of conflict for some people, the rates of suicide and attempts at suicide are higher than average for this group.

You are not alone.

Attempting suicide is not the answer, but talking to someone is.

Ask for help.

This is a good time to seek some counselling so that you can make sense of your situation and make plans for managing it. There are telephone counselling services available, or you may find a counsellor in your area that you can see face-to-face. For Australia, see the *AIFS* website[94] for more information.

It is helpful to be able to come out to your family and friends at a time that is appropriate for you. It is important to be able to understand how your family may react and to prepare yourself for that reaction. It is to be hoped that your family are supportive and accept you as you are, and of course, your friends too. You may tell those people that are more likely to support you first. You may also consider how much you accept yourself as a sexual being having the identity and orientation that you have. The more comfortable you are with the situation the better able you will be to withstand any ensuing conflict. This might mean that you sit with the idea for a little while before you start coming out to others. Or perhaps only tell a select few.

TRANSGENDER

For transgender kids the situation in Australia is better now than it used to be. Provided the situation is picked up before puberty, hormone blockers can be prescribed so that puberty is delayed. Assessment by two psychiatrists is required for hormone treatment and gender reassignment to take place.

Recently, a full sitting of the Family Court made a ruling that the court is no longer involved in the process granting young transgender kids experiencing gender dysphoria the right to gender-affirming hormone treatment. This will make transitioning a less costly and more humane process for young people.

It is important for you to accept your own sexuality and sexual identity, as well as that of others. Your sexuality and sexual identity are part of who you are, deep down, and require acceptance. And if you accept your own sexuality and sexual identity then others have the right for you to accept theirs too.

CONSENT

No one has the right to abuse you.

No one has the right to do anything that you do not consent to.

Consent is a very important aspect of any type of sexual behaviour. Whether you are male or female you need to gain verbal consent to whatever you are intending to do or proposing to do with a partner— and if at any stage you get a 'no' or any word or behaviour that might indicate a negative then you need to stop what you are doing immediately.

It doesn't matter if you got a verbal agreement previously or not. It is important to take notice of the change of agreement, because legally you have no leg to stand on if you continue and, even more importantly, you are violating the other person's rights as a human being.

You would like your rights to be respected, so ensure that you also afford those rights to others.

To put the above in an easy-to-understand way, we can think about consent as being equivalent to making a cup of tea. Consent is far more nuanced, and this analogy doesn't consider disability, consent given while incapacitated (for instance, if the person agrees but they are drunk and therefore not in a position to make a clear decision). However, it gives a basic outline that is useful to follow.

CONSENT AND TEA

If you ask someone if they would like a cup of tea, and they say 'no thank you', then don't make them tea.

If you ask someone if they would like a cup of tea, and they say 'yes please', then you can make them a cup of tea. However, if they change their mind and don't want to drink it, don't force them to drink it.

If someone is unconscious, don't make them tea. Unconscious people don't want tea—even if they said they wanted tea while they were still conscious. If someone is unconscious, make sure they are safe. And forget all about tea.

The same thing applies to sex and any kind of sexual behaviour, no matter what it is.

The legal age of consent in Australia varies among the States, generally being 16 years old. Legally, anyone under that age cannot give consent. You are liable to be charged and convicted of sexual intercourse without consent of a minor if you have sex with a minor. This is commonly referred to as rape, although that term is no longer in use in the court of law.

If your partner is over the age of consent, but doesn't consent to a sexual act then you can be charged with similar offences. When it comes to any sexual act, respect the rights of others, stick to the consent rules, and think of the long-term consequences, and you will have healthy sexual relationships—and not get into trouble with the law.

Only you have the right to allow or prohibit behaviours that involve you and your body. This includes sexting. This is another boundary you can put into place for yourself and in your dating relationships.

In general, it will be wise to practice responsible and mindful behaviour when taking, sharing, and storing images on your phone, and the internet. If you are mindful of the fact that the internet is permanent, are cautious in sharing your personal information, are respectful of others' privacy, and consider carefully what you are sharing and take consent into account – both yours and others', this will be a good start. Sometimes situations and relationships change and along with this, emotions and feelings change too. Considering such a possibility may be useful in your decision making.

SEXUAL CONSENT

Consent in any sexual encounter is crucial. You can withdraw consent at any time.

If your partner respects you then they will stop. If they don't stop, they can be charged with sexual intercourse without consent or sexual assault.

Between two consenting people, sex can be inspiring, rejuvenating and satisfying. In any case, it is important to think about any possible consequences of your behaviour. Birth control needs to be discussed with your partner, and the use of condoms is a good idea.

Condoms stop sexually transmitted infections (STIs) such as chlamydia, which can make females infertile. Gonorrhoea and syphilis are on the rise in current times and these are sexually transmitted diseases that are very unpleasant, although treatable with penicillin. Gonorrhoea may be asymptomatic (that is, no symptoms), but may have discharges, and otherwise this can be a sight-threatening disease. There can be complications such as pelvic inflammatory disease, rashes, abscess in glands, and pustules may also develop. Syphilis has a 50% likelihood of being asymptomatic. However, symptoms may occur, and firstly, there can be an ulcer or ulcers at the site of entry, which may be unnoticed. The incubation period is between 10 and 90 days, (around 3 weeks on average). This stage is highly infectious. After 6 weeks, the second stage begins. Here, there are systemic (affects body functions) symptoms that you will notice. These include fever, headaches, lymph nodes often swell and enlarge, skin rashes are very common. Neurological signs may include vision changes, head and cranial issues such as meningitis or deafness. This stage is extremely infectious to sexual partners and to a foetus. These progressions are still only within the first stage of syphilis, and the disease will progress further if you do not notice. Even the symptoms may resolve themselves, but it is important to seek treatment early rather than continuing to ignore them[95].

Another sexually transmitted disease is HIV (Human Immunodeficiency Virus). Although having better options for treatment now, it is still prevalent in many places and there is a need for care and awareness, whether or not you are queer. Between 2013 and 2017 there was a 25% increase in notifications of HIV infection through heterosexual contact[96]. Thus, it is not just a need to be careful for mem who have sex with men, those that inject drugs, sex workers, and Aboriginal and Torres Strait Islanders, but for everyone.

If you are young and sexually active, then visiting an STI clinic regularly is a good option, and having your partner provide you with a clean bill of health from a STI clinic ensures you are both keeping each other's best interests at heart (don't just trust their word for it, have them present the receipt).

The safest way to treat any partner is to always use condoms. If your partner complains that they don't like using condoms because the feeling is more limited, the answer to this is that they will last longer and can get satisfaction from knowing they are satisfying you.

Family planning clinics are a good option for finding out the different kinds of contraception to use so you are in charge of your body. Sometimes family planning and sexual health screening is provided at the same place, so explore what is available in your area.

If you are male, you need to have some say in birth control too. It is much better for children to be planned by both parents, who have discussed everything together.

If you want a child and you are quite young, think about what this might mean for your life. Work out if it is the right time or whether waiting a couple of years might be better.

It's much better to plan and to discuss with your partner, because they are involved, whether you like it or not.

HEALTHY SEXUAL RELATIONSHIPS

In a healthy sexual relationship, you can keep safe boundaries between fantasy and reality.

Any fantasies that you indulge in when you are masturbating are best kept to those times.

If you find you need to fantasise when you are making love with a partner, then recognise it for what it is: just a fantasy.

Most importantly, if you have a healthy relationship, hopefully you are having fun.

When you are fulfilling your lust with someone you love, then you make a deep emotional connection with them.

It is a good idea to sit down and define where your boundaries are in relation to sex. You may wish to do this independently or with your partner.

Your boundaries will be related to what you like and dislike, and what you are willing to give and receive. Define your boundaries and plan beforehand so that it will be easier to recognise when those boundaries are being crossed and you are being taken advantage of.

If you do decide to work out your boundaries independently, you could also have a conversation with your partner and define your boundaries with them, once you are clear in your own mind, and you could talk about your partner's boundaries too. Once you have both talked about the activities you like and dislike then you will be on the same page, and your sex life will improve.

In a healthy sexual relationship, sex is only a part of the relationship. You need to enjoy each other's company and spend time together doing things you both like.

You can also socialise together, with others or just the two of you.

A big part of the relationship should be communication. Communication is the key to a healthy relationship, since you need to understand each other, and you do this through healthy communication, in whatever mode this is[97].

See the previous chapter for more.

UNHEALTHY RELATIONSHIPS

How do you recognise an unhealthy relationship?

A relationship is unhealthy when one person feels that they are being taken advantage of, when their personal boundaries are being crossed and when they feel used and/or abused.

An unhealthy relationship exists when there is violence, psychological, or emotional abuse.

When you are being controlled by your partner, when you do not have the freedom to be yourself, when sex is the primary activity, when you are being criticised all the time, being put down—either in front of others, when the two of you are alone, or both; these are all indications that should make you think about whether you want to remain in such a relationship.

While some of these situations may be easier to manage than others, they are all signs of at least an unhealthy situation. You are, after all, two different people in a relationship and you should each accept the other person as an individual who is different from you. There is an intersection where the two of you meet, and that is you as a couple.

This is where you communicate, agree on decisions, talk together, and do things together. But apart from the two of you as a couple you are two unique individuals, and respect for each other should be paramount. This should be shown by respecting each other's personal boundaries. Situations like the ones discussed here actually break personal boundaries.

Sex and power are interrelated. If you feel that your relationship has an unequal balance in favour of one person, then explore what this means and think about whether it is really about power. Some people exploit others, and the feeling of being the more powerful one in the relationship may be a buzz for them. It may be important to seek change when you can.

Domestic violence is related primarily to violence in the home. This includes physical violence, sexual violence, emotional or psychological abuse, and coercive control (this includes limiting access to finances, monitoring movements, and isolating from friends and family).

Social attitudes and beliefs still appear to excuse these behaviours to some extent, despite the higher public awareness over the last few years, and with Grace Tame being the 2021 Australian of The Year.

The statistical estimate is that 20% of Australians have experienced some kind of domestic violence (from 2016 PSS Survey)[98].

The pandemic increased violence, particularly towards women, due to the family situation of being in lockdown and restricted movements being in place. Almost two thirds of the women surveyed who experienced physical or sexual violence reported that it had either started or escalated around the time of the pandemic[99].

Digital and technological opportunities that now exist for tracking someone's movements have increased the prevalence of this form of monitoring. Coercive control in the context of domestic violence is illegal in some countries overseas, including England, Ireland and Scotland[100].

Leaving an unhealthy relationship can present difficulties. The decision to part ways may not come easily, considering the shared memories, possessions, and history between both individuals.

If you still have feelings for your partner, you might consider giving them the opportunity to address their behaviour through relationship counselling. Whether this approach proves effective may be an indication of a willingness to change. However, if you have previously requested change and they have not responded it may be necessary to consider your options seriously.

Engaging in individual counselling can be helpful in gathering your strength and formulating plans and finding the support out in the community that is available.

Where there is domestic violence and coercive control the most dangerous time may be when you are planning and intending to leave. Seeking local support and making sure you are protected in the process of leaving a domestic violence relationship is crucial. If you haven't been with them long, you may have an easier time making a cleaner break compared to having a long-term relationship.

Even so, it is important to understand the possible ramifications of the consequences of your leaving the relationship. You know your partner best, be guided by this knowledge and how you know they are likely to react[101]. Discussion with your partner is preferable but may not always be advisable or appropriate.

You could check out the legal situation, and check the shelters in your area if you are going to need one. Preparation is a good thing. Plan the easiest way of leaving.

You might need to find other accommodation. Moving out your possessions will also be necessary. It is easier if you can move out, rather than getting your partner to move out. But each situation is unique and will depend upon circumstances.

HISTORICAL SEXUAL ABUSE

If you have suffered sexual abuse in the past, it will be necessary for you to redefine yourself. You can choose to be a survivor rather than a victim.

If you continually bring the subject up, particularly in context of being unable to achieve things you would like to achieve, you may be defining yourself as a victim.

Choose instead to be a survivor who has healthy boundaries. So set a boundary for others to show respect to you.

Do not let others take advantage of you and speak out when you notice this happening.

Be assertive.

Set boundaries that allow you to care for yourself. Do things to nurture yourself on a regular basis. Let others know when they are abusing your boundaries and give them consequences for crossing them. It might be three different actions that you tell them you will put into place.

You can create your own consequences, but you need to tell them what will happen. Thus, you need to be assertive. See the chapter on assertiveness for further information.

It is certainly the case that any kind of trauma does change the brain[102]. However, this does not mean that you cannot find your unique self-healing pathway to peace and purpose.

It is important to understand that talk alone may continue to retraumatise you.

To find your pathway to healing, doing something different with your memories, and engaging in actual processes that help to change your emotions, beliefs, thoughts, and perceptions around your past experiences is going to be important.

See later chapters for more information on healing trauma.

We cannot change what happened in the past, but we can change how we feel and think about it.

GENERAL RELATIONSHIP ASPECTS

It is ok to cut ties with a partner, whatever length your relationship is. Whether you stay or go really depends on your own needs.

Relationships that are healthy for you would likely provide some freedom for you to grow within the relationship, and for the two of you to grow together as well.

If you find this is not happening, and the relationship is not meeting your needs then it is totally up to you to exit.

DATING

In the dating game, while you are exploring your sexuality and possibly having short-term partners, you may come across "ghosting" and "orbiting".

Ghosting occurs when someone you have been communicating with, or possibly even dating, suddenly no longer responds to any attempt at communication.

Orbiting is similar; however, the person continues to engage with your social media activity by liking your posts and watching your stories, but does not read or respond to direct messages.

Online dating and communication through social media and via text has made ghosting more prevalent and has created the possibility for orbiting to exist.

If you are a person who regularly ghosts or orbits others, have a think about what this kind of behaviour is saying about you. Essentially, you are not taking responsibility for your choice of action, you are not respecting the people you interact with, and you are not respecting yourself. In any communication, it is important to see others as equal to you, to discuss your decisions honestly and in person where possible.

If there is absolutely no danger to you, then discussing the situation and your decision to stop communicating gives some respect to the other person. Feedback is often helpful for others, and it might also be helpful for you. Everyone can learn through relationships.

Where you are the person being ghosted, consider what you have learnt from this relationship, write down what aspects you have found you do not want in a partner, and those you do. This is something you can take forward.

Whether this is from a partner or friend, allow yourself the time to create your own feedback, come to some assessment, and allow it to be accepted in your mind and heart.

If this is difficult for any reason, then perhaps you could seek help from a professional.

> For any relationship difficulty or issue, it does come down to trusting yourself and trusting and listening to those around you who love you and who have your best interests at heart.

SEXUAL HARASSMENT

Where you are being sexually harassed outside of the home environment, by your boss or someone who has greater power over you, then you may need to be quite careful. If this is being carried out by co-workers, then the course of action you take will, to some extent, depend on the particular circumstances, and will include factors such as whether you feel able to stand up for yourself and what kind of harassment it is—so for instance, if there is a discriminatory component to the harassment, it may strengthen your case and make it easier to resolve the situation.

In any case, it is important to get support from a professional outside of your work situation who may be able to help you think through the situation and deal with it in the best way possible. Many employers, and particularly larger companies and organisations, have an Employee Assistance Program (EAP), which may allow you to have a number of counselling sessions free of charge. Additionally, there are some government and outside organisations that would be able to provide advice to you.

SUMMARY

- Communicate with your family, and ask for help if you need it.

- Communicate with your partner and ensure consent in any sexual behaviour or act.

- Have healthy relationships with others and recognise when you are in an unhealthy relationship. Leaving may be the best option in the latter case.

- Accept both your own and others' sexuality.

- Treat yourself and others with respect and communicate clearly and honestly.

- By taking these steps you can start creating a healthy attitude to sex and at the same time, keep yourself safe.

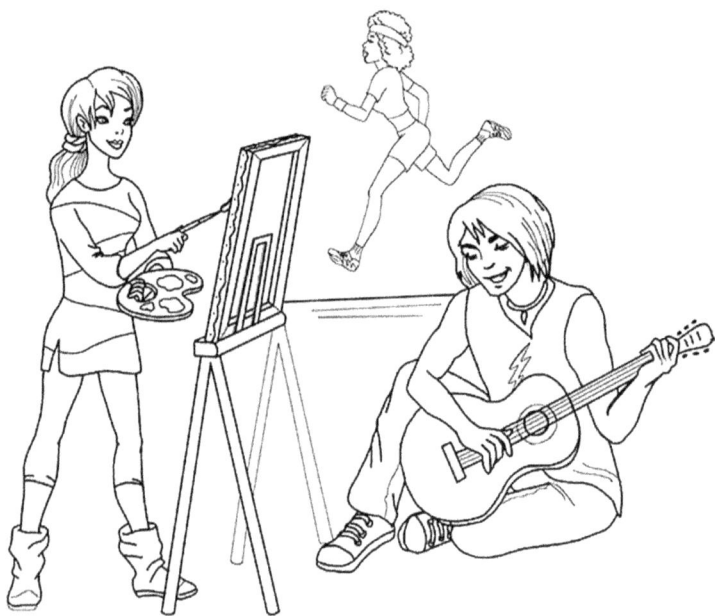

CHAPTER 6

INTERESTS AND HOBBIES

Hobbies and interests expand your learning and capacity for growth

Hobbies and interests can continue over a lifetime. They may be something that you like to do when you have some free time. You may set aside some time every week to walk, hike, or cycle. It doesn't matter if an interest just remains something that you do regularly. There is no rule that says something you like needs to become a career. Sometimes it can. Otherwise, it just stays as an interest.

Hobbies and interests are certainly good for your mental health. They provide rest, relaxation, and exercise, and can be very beneficial for your general heath.

Whether it is something that you do by yourself or with others, such activities provide time for *you*, which means that they are part of self-care. If you can look after yourself then this means you are more capable of looking after others too.

Engaging in hobbies and interesting activities refreshes your mind and helps you to gain a new perspective on life. Engaging in hobbies is one important area where you can find freedom and fulfilment, and presents the opportunity to feed and nurture yourself. Spend time on things that you like to do whenever you are able. You will be glad when you do.

What this means is that hobbies and interests may continue over a short period of time or a lifetime and provide an enjoyable way to engage your attention and free time. They don't need to turn into careers; rather, they can be pursued for personal enjoyment, relaxation and satisfaction.

Additionally, they are avenues for gaining new perspectives on your life and nurturing yourself. When you engage in activities that you genuinely enjoy, a sense of fulfilment is created, as well as that of freedom. Pursuing such interests can lead to personal growth, and provides a more complete understanding of yourself and has potential benefits in other areas of life.

POSITIVE EFFECTS

There are often unique opportunities to discover skills and develop your talents when you are following your heart and applying yourself to new interests. Through trying different activities, you are exploring interests and passions that may eventually lead to finding innate and previously unknown talents. These talents may or may not become career paths. Whether or not they do does not matter because engaging in them can be personally rewarding no matter what.

Other positive effects of engaging in hobbies are numerous, from boosting self-esteem, self-confidence and feelings of competence to fostering transferable skills you can apply in other areas of life and out into the wider world.

Transferable skills are those skills and knowledge that you accumulate that are useful in all areas of life and across many different situations. These may include such things as attention to detail, concentration, focus, organisational skills, leadership ability, strong teamwork, communication skills, knowledge, and strategic ability. Transferable skills may help you secure a place at university, where you may have gained knowledge and interview skills through school and your hobbies. This might help you to find more clarity on what you want to do. Then there are the specific skills that are related to your particular hobby or interest that may apply to other areas.

Additionally, some hobbies, such as sport, can contribute to your physical fitness and general health too. Involvement in sporting activities provides opportunity for exercise and teamwork experience. It doesn't necessarily need to lead anywhere such as a professional sporting career. Finding and developing a number of plans, including a number of different options to follow, with one of those at least being a fallback position will be beneficial in the long term. Overall, planning for the long term can be an extremely good strategy.

While some hobbies may lead to careers, it is beneficial to remember that you are not solely defined by your talents and skills. It is totally your choice as to whether you follow a path that involves your talent or skill. *It is your life and your choice.*

The decision to turn a hobby into your profession should be a personal choice. Following your heart and your passions is more important than external recognition or success when this is your preference. It is totally up to you how you engage in your hobby. It can be a life-long interest which you engage with in your leisure time, you may just do it for a period of time, or it can turn into a career eventually. This might happen at a much later date. Early interests and hobbies can be revived at any time when you choose to do so. If you have an innate talent for it and you are passionate about it later, and it appeals to you, then it may indicate a positive career move then.

A hobby may be an important addition in your life, or it might build on what you are already doing so it adds to an existing framework. This situation may mean that you are being aided in your main work or career by what you are doing in your leisure time as a hobby.

When your hobby or interest is more social or team oriented than a solo activity, then the social interaction enables friendships and your social circle is likely to widen. Building relationships with others is what humans are built to do and because social support is and contact is so important in our lives, this is another major benefit in helping yourself thrive and maintain your health and wellbeing on all levels. It is helpful for giving you a sense of being more connected in life, belonging, and having relationships with like-minded people.

In the process, you may learn new things, find out new information, and gaining numerous skills that you may not otherwise learn, including team skills, where appropriate. Becoming involved in the wider community outside of your family and school means that you become a more multidimensional person. By engaging in a hobby that holds your interest, you are expressing who you are.

This has positive health benefits; not only for physical health, but for mental health as well. You may find a sense of freedom in engaging in your hobby or activity and find that time just flies by. This is the space of being "in flow", when you are absolutely present in the now and you are engaging in what you love. This is what you are looking for when you engage in your hobby, and this feeling can inform your decisions.

SOME NEGATIVE SITUATIONS

Negative situations may arise when hobbies or activities are forced upon you when you are not really interested. This can lead to resentment and disinterest. You could end up resenting the amount of time the activity takes, and also resentment may build up towards whoever instigated it. It is only when you also choose to do it that the negatives won't outweigh the positives.

Where you have unfulfilled desires of engaging in a particular hobby or activity due to circumstances there are options that can arise later. Perhaps the costs were prohibitive or somehow you were unable to engage in your interests. If this happens when young or is occurring now, then, should you be of the same mind later, you can choose to set a goal then, and go about achieving it. It is never too late to try.

The circumstances need to come together so that everything is in place for you to reach your goal. Sometimes, the options you want may not be available later and the time for your exact desired outcome may have passed. You may however be able to find a good alternative activity that fulfils at least a part of your unfulfilled desires if this is the case. There may be other ways that you can be fulfilled in your interest area too. It is a matter of exploration and discovery.

For example, if you are too old to reach competition level in dance or sport, then it might be possible to become a coach or teacher, or simply to enjoy the mental and physical health benefits and social aspects of participating dance or sport.

Similarly, where you are not supported in your desire to engage in a hobby or interest when young, then this may have a different impact on you. It may mean that you need to come up with other alternatives that may be supported which are still close to your heart. It depends on your individual circumstances and your particular interest. There are always alternatives to explore.

START OUT EARLY

Exploring talents and creativity is crucial. This is the case not only in the area of potential career paths related to your talents, but in hobbies and interests too. Nurturing and developing in a number of areas when young can be empowering and enhance your decision-making abilities in relation to both career moves and leisure activities.

While young, carry out this exploration process. Try as many things as you can that you can imagine yourself doing that could become hobbies or sporting interests. Hopefully, your primary caregivers are helping or guiding you with attending classes, games, and so on, and allowing you to follow your interests and passions.

Depending on what it is and how skilled you become at it, it may become an even bigger part of your life. Think about the hobbies you had earlier or those you are considering pursuing now. Whether present or past, what you are doing or have done may help you sort out what you like and what you aren't really interested in. The question is then what are you really keen on? Have some interests lasted and, if so, how do you feel about them?

TRAVEL IN YOUR MIND

Hopefully, reading books is on your list of hobbies and interests. Reading books helps you learn about the world, increases your vocabulary, helps spelling, and provides entertainment. If books are interesting for you then there are a number of roads you could take. You could join a book club, learn about particular subjects and topics, or learn about various countries before you go travelling. Books also increase your creativity, imagination, and usually help your thinking ability, as well as providing information that can be applied in different situations. The fact that you are reading this book means you are interested in learning about things!

TRAVEL IN REALITY

Travelling offers educational opportunities to learn about different cultures, and lifestyles, to see different landscapes and environments. This all contributes to personal growth and broadening your horizons. Safety measures and research is essential prior to travelling to an unfamiliar place, so check out the appropriate information on trusted websites or other sources.

Additionally, it is a good idea to inform yourself on local customs and laws so that you don't fall into trouble in a strange place. Through ensuring you understand the visa requirements and safety measures, you will have a smooth and more welcome travel experience.

CREATIVITY EXPLORATION

Nurture your creativity in any area, and explore those things you are passionate about that can lead to fulfilling hobbies and potential career paths. Music, art, theatre, film, writing, performing, acting, drawing, singing, dancing: there are just so many options for talented people in these arenas. Investigate options and think carefully and creatively about your talents and how these may be expressed for positive outcomes. Diving deep into this may open up doors to exciting possibilities.

SELF-ASSESSMENT

You can make a list of all the things you have tried, and note which ones you are still continuing, and which ones you love to do. If you have a natural talent or skill in what you love then make a note of this too. This is important and may well indicate a possible career path, whether sooner or later.

Interests and hobbies may change as you grow older. Interests are not necessarily fixed at any age. Because interests change over time you can become more fulfilled by engaging in hobbies and activities that are appropriate at the time.

It is a great idea to be involved in sporting activities at all stages of life. It is a good source of exercise, and if it's a team sport then you develop skills as a team player. Even if you are only involved for a few years, you will gain benefits.

NEW DIRECTIONS

When you are willing to try new activities, you are steering yourself in new directions. The outcome is unknown and you are spreading your sphere of influence. It doesn't really matter what the ultimate outcome or result will be, because the process of engaging in the activity is what counts.

The process is likely to open up your world and help you expand your mind.

New learning creates new pathways in your brain, and this all goes towards your growth as a person. Whether you take it a lot further or not, the process is important. Nothing you learn is ever wasted, as it all goes towards becoming part of who you are. Follow your enthusiasm and you will find whatever you are interested in.

Taking the time to consolidate is also helpful in the learning process.

Allow yourself to plateau for a while as you practice what you have learnt. Over time, the new behaviours will become a more intrinsic part of you; they will become automatic. The new thinking will become more familiar, and you'll be able to engage in the activity with a greater level of freedom, as you will have internalised a number of the skills required to participate without needing to consciously think about what to do.

Hobbies and interests play a significant role in personal growth, self-expression, and mental wellbeing. They offer many benefits from relaxation and physical health to potential career opportunities. It is good to explore as many of your interests as possible, to nurture talents and creativity and to find those activities that bring joy and fulfillment all through your life. Whether they remain hobbies or eventually turn into careers, hobbies enrich your life and contribute to a well-rounded, multidimensional personality.

SUMMARY

- Explore a variety of interests and hobbies and find the ones that you enjoy.

- Think about whether your hobbies and interests might lead to possible career options or remain short term or lifelong activities.

- Plan some time to spend on your interests during the week. It helps rest and relaxation, and mental health as well as recharging your energy levels.

- Think about expressing your talents and interests throughout your life so your life is enhanced.

- By taking these steps, you will be on your way to having great interests and hobbies that will continue to sustain you throughout your life.

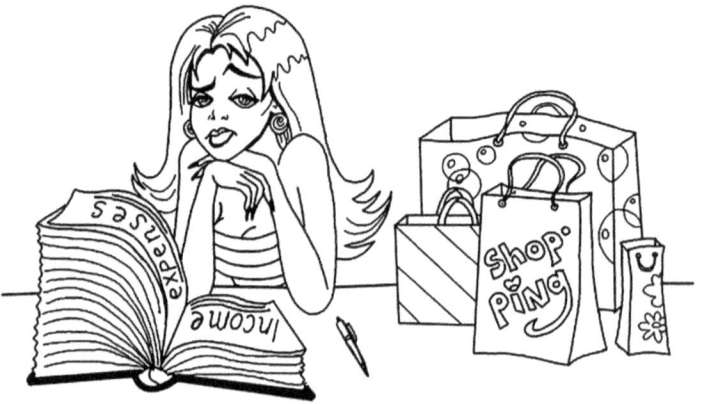

CHAPTER 7

FINANCES

What is your relationship like with money?

Given how our society and the world economy is organised, we need to accept that money is necessary. We need money to survive.

With this in mind, what can you do to arrange your finances in a way that is helpful to you? Money is both symbolic and physical, but on another level, it is just energy.

To delve deeper, money is a symbol and how we learn about that symbol can influence our experience with it. As a result, the beliefs and attitudes you learned when you were a child about money, may, to a large extent, affect the experience you have with money in your life [103].

For instance, if you have a scarcity mentality you believe that life's resources are like a finite pie. This would mean that money is a limited resource. What this means is that if others have money, then there is less for you, and you focus on that to the exclusion of other things[104]. Whereas if you have an abundance mentality (where you have a mindset that resources like money are unlimited), then you may be much more relaxed and less stressed in the same situation. There is a balance here.

If you believe that you will be financially comfortable then you may find that you are more able to live within your means. After all, all you need is more money coming in than going out. You may need some self-discipline, but it will be worth it in the long run.

BUDGETING

Financial literacy is extremely important, because there are so many traps out there that make it much more difficult to navigate if you are unaware of problems and issues around money management.

A budget is an important feature of your financial arrangements. It can help you to portion your money to the crucial expenses and help you to manage your money overall.

Everyone has expenses as well as outgoings, you hopefully also have some money coming in.

It is important to make an account of your money. As part of this process, it helps to record all the incoming and outgoing transactions as they occur. There are apps and various online programs available now that will help in this regard.

If you record everything for a few months you can then work out your averages per month. Additionally, you will know what your biggest expenditures are, and you can then look at how you might reduce your spending so that you can save more.

You can probably do this research retrospectively too, by looking through your online banking transactions and work out the totals for all expenses and income.

It is good if you can save some money. It might be helpful if you can save at least $2,500 so that you have some money in case of emergencies.

After you have worked out your average spending, you can make a list of your wants and needs. In the "needs" column you would have things like rent, food, bills.

In the "wants" column you would probably have things like the money you spend on socialising, and other things you like but don't really need. In this way you can assess where your budget is up to, and whether you are able to save money by perhaps cutting out some of the spending on things you want, rather than need.

Nowadays, it is important to have a smartphone. If you already have one, and it is working well for your needs, think seriously about keeping it rather than upgrading to the latest one.

Shop around and wait for sales, if you decide to buy a new phone investigate all options in relation to pre-paid plans or buying the phone as you go (so you are paying the phone off and also paying the monthly fee).

Sometimes it may be cheaper to buy a phone outright from one place or platform, and then find a good and cheap plan that suits your needs from a different provider.

Take your time and don't rush it.

Investigate all options and ask others, and make as many enquiries as possible.

The more money you can save, the better off you will be in the long run.

You will probably have at least a monthly phone bill that you need to take into account in your budget.

From whatever income you get you need to set aside a certain amount for living expenses. The most important of these is your rent or housing, followed by food, phone, utility bills such as gas and electricity, and transport costs—whether a car, bicycle, motorbike, or bus/train/ferry pass. After all this you need to provide for other expenses that you might pay in cash or by card, such as for socialising.

On a smartphone there are a number of budgeting apps available that you can use. Investigate them and choose the best one for you.

There are some good books on how to become financially savvy. See *Rich Dad Poor Dad*[105] and *The Barefoot Investor*[106] for a start.

SOCIAL SECURITY

It is difficult to afford everything if you are on Social Security payments, and you probably have to rely on savings—if you have any. If you are on Social Security payments and can keep within that limit, you may be making a number of sacrifices. Investigate charity options, such as food banks or local neighbourhood houses that may be able to help you manage better.

LIMITED BUDGET

If you are employed, full-time or part-time, it is still a really good idea to set a budget and stick with it. You may be able to save some money sooner if you do this, so you can have a better life.

If you have a limited budget, it's a good idea to watch debt. It can be more affordable to pay bills monthly rather than yearly, for example car registration and insurance. There may be a facility to enable gas and electricity bills to be paid monthly or fortnightly too. Investigate options such as these, and if they work for you then you can set them up.

UNEMPLOYED OR NOT

If you are unemployed then you are likely to be living hand-to-mouth, and the only long-term goal you can think about is to find employment of whatever kind possible, but preferably in an area where you have experience or interest. It's very tough being unemployed, no matter when this occurs in your life. It is particularly demoralising when no one will even give you the opportunity to show them what you can do.

If your money is low, it is good to preserve as much of it as possible, rather than spending what you don't have. There are a number of traps for the consumer that you need to be aware of.

Firstly, there are advertisements for companies that allow you to borrow small amounts of money without credit checks. These are generally called "payday loan companies". It is not a good idea to get caught in their clutches.

The interest rates they charge are beyond comprehension (47.8% to 65.3%) and you might end up getting multiple loans to pay off previous loans.

For instance, if you were to borrow $300 with these interest rates, you would be paying back $443 to $579.

Even if you are optimistic and believe that you can pay the first loan back without any trouble, circumstances may intervene and mean that you get caught up in the treadmill of multiple loans. The majority of people who use payday loan companies take out multiple loans.

As with any loan, it is important that you do your research and find out the interest rates. Don't just accept that you will be able to afford the repayments.

Payday loan companies do not stipulate the number of months or years the loan will run for. It is advisable to avoid these companies. The same applies to offers from finance companies as they can be loan sharks.

There are also companies that offer personal loans. Again, do your research. Check the interest rate, and work out how much money you'd be paying back overall.

Ensure that you are getting the best deal if you are after a personal loan. Shop around for the best deal. Think about credit unions as well as the usual high street banks. Question whether you really need a personal loan. You may be better off saving up the money. Perhaps you can delay what you want to do with the money. Look at your circumstances properly.

BUY NOW PAY LATER

In recent years, there has been a shake-up in the credit card industry and companies offer options of "buy now, pay later". While this is appealing, since there is an interest-free period provided you are making the payments, there is a trap here if you overextend yourself and are unable to afford them.

If you lose track of what you have already put on this scheme, then you may end up needing to get loans from the payday lenders mentioned above, or just end up with so much debt you land yourself in trouble. If you do end up with multiple debts, ask for help.

Firstly, you can approach the company you owe money to. Secondly, check out the Australian Government *Money Smart* website[107]. There is free financial counselling and advice available too.

In any case, whether you are this far down the debt road or not, it is important to record every transaction so that you can keep track of it all. If you do keep track of all your incomes and expenses, then the good news is you can make better decisions around your spending habits and work on getting out of debt more easily.

CREDIT CARDS

Credit card debt can mount up quickly if you are not paying it off regularly. It is a good policy to only have one credit card. You should investigate the best possible interest charged and choose the lowest interest with an interest free period. Some institutions now offer better options than in the past. If you are able to pay off what you owe every month during the interest free period then you will save yourself a lot of money in the long run.

When searching for credit card providers don't be sucked in by interest free periods on balances switched over. Look more at what the *usual* interest rate is. It is a false economy to switch over for the sake of switching. Any new purchases will be charged at the going interest rate for that card. If you aren't going to be strict with yourself and just pay off the remaining balance in the next six or twelve months allotted without spending more money on your card then it will cost you a lot more.

By reining in your spending and being strict with yourself, you can get your credit card debt down to zero. Get the number of credit cards you have down to one, and pay it off monthly. Then you will be able to say that you are in control of your credit card rather than letting your spending control you.

Additionally, you could have a decision-making period involving your credit card so that you don't just make an impulsive purchase with it. For instance, you could leave your credit card in a tub of water in the freezer, so that the ice would need to melt before you can use it to make a purchase. Perhaps you could also have a policy of saying, 'no' to people who may contact you and pressure you to give money to charities or other entities. You could also work out for yourself a decision-making routine around online shopping.

You may need to write a letter or email to your credit card lender and state that you want to close your credit card account. Do not get sucked in when they counter with higher limits, less interest or any other ploy. Stick to your goal and remain on track so that you can close the account properly. Do not just cut up your card, because payments may continue to accrue. You need to stop any regular payments that go onto your credit card before you close the account. Get the balance down to zero and then close the account through the bank or other authority. Then do the same with your other credit cards, until you are left with only one.

The credit card you keep should have the lowest interest rate with an interest free period, or at least be cheaper overall. Then you will need to keep an account of what you put on it so that you can afford to pay it off every month. In this way, you will be on top of your spending.

Don't forget that the money that you put on your credit card or on buy now, pay later is money *you don't have*. That is why it's called credit.

SUPERANNUATION

Although your employer is obliged to put money in your superannuation account for you, if you can contribute as well it will be worthwhile. Do not put it off, because you may regret it later. You will need a lot of money in your super account so that you are able to live comfortably in your retirement. Life can be unpredictable, but it is best to plan for your future, whatever that may look like.

From the financial year of 2017/2018 superannuation contributions are tax deductible in Australia (check out the situation in your area). It is even more economical and helpful in the long-term to make your own contributions to your super. It helps to consolidate your super money so that it is all in one superannuation fund—which can be done through the Australian Tax Office—and to do so in an industry super fund.

Investigate your industry super fund, especially in terms of fees and insurance.

You can organise to have work cover and accident insurance as well. Compare fees with Australian Super Fund, which is an industry super fund.

It may be better to nominate the super fund you want your employer to contribute to on your behalf, then you don't have to keep on rolling small balances over in the future. Whether you have full or part-time employment, your employer should be contributing to your superannuation on your behalf.

Some employers have dodged this obligation in the past, so it may be useful to check with your superannuation fund to see if contributions are being made. If you find you are being cheated, then go to your trade union and complain. You can also check whether you are being paid the correct hourly rate. Sometimes, due to the complexity of the payroll system and differences in sorting through the legislation, employers may end up paying less than is required by law. The fact that it may be a genuine oversight does not excuse them from their obligations as an employer. Whether it is intentional or unintentional, if you think you are not receiving the correct amount of money, it is certainly worthwhile checking. It's important to know that you can put in a complaint to the Fair Work Ombudsman and to know your rights.

In the circumstance where you are contributing to your super and generally paying your way in the world, then you could think about saving some money towards future investments in your life. Banks and building societies usually have online savings accounts that attract a higher interest rate than everyday accounts. You could save a certain amount each week or fortnight into one of these accounts. You can also investigate the investing strategies of your super fund, some offer options to invest in volatile options that may make you money faster but at a much higher risk.

SAVING MONEY

If you have a dedicated account for your savings, it will be easier to prove that you have a good savings history for buying expensive items. See if you can save as quickly as possible. Of course, it will depend on your income and any current expenses that you need to account for.

You might need to sacrifice some nights out on the town in order to save faster.

It may be worthwhile to do this, though. You could try going out with your friends to places that are less expensive or even free, such as going to the beach or to a park.

Another less expensive option is to socialise at your friend's homes, and share the cost of food and drink. This is far cheaper than going out. It is all a matter of negotiation and creativity. Going out and socialising doesn't always have to entail consuming large amounts of alcohol, getting drunk, and spending lots of money.

HOME OWNERSHIP

Since the price of a house in today's market is more out of reach for first home buyers, than ever, many more young people are renting for longer, and finding it much more difficult to get into the market in the first place.

The difficulty with this is that paying rent is an expense that is not flowing into an asset—it simply keeps a roof over your head.

The private rental market is expensive and this means that renting a relatively decent place makes it hard to save a reasonable amount towards your own home.

Two salaries may work better together in this respect, but it is a good idea to come to an arrangement about how you split or merge your money.

If you are still living with your parents, you have a better deal. This is your best opportunity to save money. If you have enough savings, it may be more beneficial to purchase an investment property, and when you have enough equity (outright ownership percentage) use this value to purchase your own home. Depending on the property market and the location, some young people discipline themselves to spending and put their money to good debt.

Generally speaking, home ownership is considered to be good debt because it is an investment. If you can get started in the property market, then the money you are paying on the capital loan and interest is very likely to give you something in return in the long run. In addition, you have a roof over your head that is stable and secure.

INVESTMENT PORTFOLIOS

Another example of good debt is an investment portfolio. It is important to assess the risk of what you are investing in. If you are investing in shares, then go for low-risk companies, with a long track record. "Blue Chip Stocks" (these are stocks offered by large, well established and financially sound companies with good reputations) will be better to invest in at first. Never go for "sure things" just on one or two peoples' advice. In the stock market, there is never a sure thing. Especially when the 'sure things' are very risky, like cryptocurrency.

Your safe share portfolio doesn't have to be large and it can be added to as you receive a tax refund or a windfall. It is better to treat the share market as a long-term investment, rather than attempting to gain a quick return[108].

Organising a reliable accountant or broker is always worthwhile before entering into investment strategies. Be aware of Capital Gains Tax and ask questions, always ask questions!

GOAL SETTING

If you don't have any long-term plans then you are likely to stay in the same situation, going from week to week. This way will not get you anywhere. It is helpful to set yourself some short, medium, and long-term goals in a number of areas of life.

You could have a career goal, a relationship goal, and a savings goal. One of your goals may be to buy a house. This would certainly be a long-term goal, and you could set yourself up with a savings plan in order to achieve this goal.

If you have at least two long-term goals, and ensure that you are taking action to achieve them, you will find that you make progress towards your goals. It is important to take a long-term view and to reflect every now and then on your progress, so that you may make changes to your goal, your strategies or the actions that you are taking. If you are interested in finding out more about money and the best ways to manage what you do, there is a good book by Scott Pape, called *Barefoot Kids*[109].

Short and medium-term goals are also good to have, because then you will feel that you are making progress as you achieve them. If you have a savings plan then you could set some short-term goals of saving $500, then $1,000, and so on, so the amount of time between achieving your short-term goals is not so great, and you feel as though you are getting somewhere.

You could then set a goal of $5,000 and then $10,000. These would be medium-term goals. However, achieving them will motivate you to keep on going to your long-term goal. For more on goal setting you can buy and read the chapter on goal setting from my first book, *A Practical Guide for Self Change*[110].

BUYING A CAR

If you are buying a car and you need additional funds, the best thing to do is to get organised and find out about getting a loan from a bank or credit union before you sign an agreement for finance at the car yard. If you do organise the loan beforehand, then you will find that you save a great deal of money. The finance companies associated with car yards usually have an interest rate of over 20%. Through a bank you may be able to get a much lower interest rate (perhaps 9% or thereabouts) and for a credit union it could be even lower. Generally, when buying a new car, you do have the issue of depreciation. This means that your new car is likely to be worth a lot less the minute you buy it and take it onto the road. There are of course other options. If you would prefer to pay less money and are willing to have a car that is older, the used car market is the way to go. Ensure that whatever car you buy is roadworthy, has not been in a serious accident, and have it checked by an authorized mechanic first.

MICROFINANCE

When you need to have an injection of money and you are on Social Security payments or have limited income, you could try searching for an ethical and secure microfinance company. You may have one in your area.

They provide interest free loans for people who have a specific reason for needing the money; sometimes up to $3,000. For example, if your refrigerator breaks down or if you need to fix your car, you may be eligible. Do your research and give them a call. They may also have other services available such as saving plans[111].

OPTIONS FOR SAVING MONEY

Stay away from companies that rent out furniture and household items. It is cheaper to shop at second hand stores or apply to charities for help with furniture and other items they carry. Renting any household item, no matter what it is, is going to be a lot more expensive than just buying it outright in the first instance. If you were to rent, then over the life of the rental agreement you would be likely to pay double or even triple the cost of the items at a normal retail shop.

Don't get sucked in by the cheap weekly payments—even though each individual payment is low, they go on for a long time, so that you end up paying far more than the items are worth.

If you need something, ask for advice from your friends, family, and people who are likely to know. If you tend to be impulsive about purchases, then it might be helpful to look at your buying patterns over time. You could also ask for help from a professional, particularly if your purchases relate to emotional issues.

Approach charities or second-hand shops in your local area and you may find good and useful furniture. Social media platforms, the Internet, local communities, friends, and family can be useful resources for finding resources including: cheap or free items, recommendations for reliable trades people, or exchanging goods and services such as plants, books, clothes, and household items. Many items are in good condition, and by utilising this method of acquiring furniture and other items, you are participating in sustainable living and recycling.

When it comes to clothing, "Fast Fashion" is increasingly recognised as problematic, and this, in combination with a big push to reduce landfill, means that quality over quantity is starting to be seen as the way forward.

It does not matter at all if you wear clothes more than once, it simply means that you like wearing it. Equally, when it comes to purchasing new clothing, just because something is fashionable doesn't mean that you need it. You can save a lot of money if you stay off the fashion treadmill. This mindset applies not only to clothes, but also to household items and interior decoration.

What does it matter if you aren't seen to be fashionable? There are deeper things to be concerned about. You don't need to dress like your favourite influencer or pop idol. They can do their thing (which they are often paid for), and you can do you.

Be the unique person you are. Don't let fashion rule your beliefs and ideas about peoples' worth and value. There are many more values to be concerned about, such as friendship, inclusion, love, truthfulness, and respect. Just as long as you wear what you like and it is appropriate for what you need to do in your day-to-day life, and just as long as household items work and are useful, that is all that matters.

When it comes down to it, what others think is none of your business. Just as long as *you're* happy, it is fine. Save yourself money and go for comfort and usefulness.

Every area of media is bombarding you with advertisements on how to live your life. You are never going to achieve it if you believe everything you see and hear. Because we live in a throwaway culture, opportunity shops and second-hand furniture provide great bargains. You can express yourself just as well, and often even more uniquely, through recycling and upcycling.

See it as a way of showing your creativity. Make it something fun. You don't have to spend a lot of money. You can still be stylish, chic, and express yourself on a lower budget.

When finding fresh and local produce, there are also Plant Groups, where you can swap plants; there are roadside swaps for fresh vegetables and fruit; along with community gardens and farmers markets— why not grow your own vegetables and fruit, if you have room? They can even grow well in pots and window boxes.

Find out about ways to save money. Whenever you can, ask for a discount. There is no harm in asking, and you might get it. There may be discounts offered if you are a member of a particular association or club. Find out about these, and then remember to ask for the discount. Sometimes there are flash sales, which can be helpful when you are ready for them. Mailing lists are sometimes good to subscribe to, as they may have money-saving perks, such as member-only sales.

> In summary, with every material purchase, think about how you can make consumerism work for you.

INSURANCE

When you are looking for an insurance product, do some investigation rather than just joining a company that advertises on television or social media.

Make a list of options and research online, asking questions that may sort out which will be the best for you. The importance of doing your own research cannot be underestimated.

Google different companies and explore their websites, so that you know you are finding out a wide range of companies offering the product you are looking for.

Read the fine print to see what the terms and conditions are and talk to people who know the industry. Talk to a number of people before making up your mind—it might be helpful to speak to a financial planner too.

Life insurance may be something to think about later once you begin your own family. Then your family is provided for if something happens to you. Compare products and choose the company that offers the best terms and conditions, along with a reasonable costing.

Contents insurance is also a good thing to have once you start renting, so that you are covered if something happens. Make sure you know the circumstances that are covered. For example, it would be helpful if the company covered "water events" rather than just "flooding". This would mean that something like a burst water main causing damage would give you a payout, rather than just a natural disaster.

Home and contents insurance is good once you own your home. You may need to be cautious in relation to where you may live and explore such things as flood plains and sea surges. Since climate change is now really kicking in, places on higher ground are going to be safer and more insurable over time.

Income protection is the number one personal protection insurance that you should consider to protect your income, if you're fully employed. The contributions are usually tax deductible.

Then there is trauma cover, also known as "critical illness cover", which is the cover that most people don't know much about. Trauma cover provides cover if you are diagnosed with a specified illness or injury, such as cancer or a stroke, that may have a big impact on your life.

Ask questions and have a meeting with a financial advisor. It is free if you are looking for some guidance and understanding of personal protection insurance.

MANAGING DEBT

Overall, it is good policy not to get into debt. However, if it is an asset such as a mortgage, where debt may be unavoidable, then the faster you can pay your debt off the better.

When you are paying off your credit card every month during the interest free period, this is paying off your debt. Where you are using a debit card instead of a credit card, this is also staying out of debt.

When buying a house, the lower the debt the better. See if you can pay it off faster than is required. If you pay on a weekly basis then you will pay less interest long-term, and if you pay more than the necessary amount then the extra comes off the principal that you owe. Some of the more basic home loan products have a lower interest rate, but no offset account.

If you decide on a loan that has the capacity for an offset account, this can be useful in reducing the overall interest that you pay. If there is no offset account then you are probably paying a lower rate of interest. But make sure you check this.

With a home loan account product, it can be better to leave the interest rate on variable, particularly when rates are decreasing. Where rates are increasing, then you can think about fixing your interest rate for a few years at a time. However, fixed terms rates are usually a bit higher than current interest rates, to allow for increases over time. Variable rates are often lower, so you may view these as being preferable.

However, if you want peace of mind and are not going to pay more off your mortgage than the institution requires, then fixing your rates for a few years may be appropriate.

Make sure you discuss the options available to you with your institution home loan manager. If you have fixed your home loan for three years and interest rates are rising, then you may be faced with a big jump in interest rates when that period ends. It is a good policy to provide yourself with a buffer in your own mind of a number of percentage points higher than the fixed rate you are paying. If you can still afford the higher rate, then you may be safe. The lending institutions are now doing a bit of a calculation around buffers, but you could make sure yourself before jumping in.

BUDGETING

If you set yourself a budget and manage to work out what you need, you may be able to save some money for your future.

Setting goals for your future will help you to achieve what it is you want. If you take a long-term view then you may find that you make better progress. Set one-year, five-year, and ten-year goals.

You may find that you can save money by doing things such as cooking your own food instead of buying takeaway. This may also help you to eat better and be healthier. All the little bits add up. A big saving, if you are able to afford it, is to purchase all your staples when they are on special. This means buying the cooking ingredients you use most often, such as: flour, sugar, tea, coffee, toothpaste, frozen vegetables, and tinned foods when they are at their cheapest, so that you have a replica store in the cupboard and you don't have to buy these items at full price.

This works well with cleaning and washing products too. You'll be amazed at the savings over a year. You might even be able to set aside enough for a nice holiday!

When you are shopping, whether for food, clothes or furniture, you can look for bargains. However, make sure that it's something that you need and are going to use. It's not a bargain if you don't need it—it's just a waste of money.

DEALING WITH DEBT

When you fall behind in paying off your loan, credit card, or utility bills, you may be contacted by a debt collector. If you disregard the debt collector and do not respond reasonably to them, then they may sue you. This means that the matter will go to court. If you disregard this, then it is likely that a judgement will be made against you.

It is better in the long run to contact the providers of the loan, credit card, or utility and enter into a payment plan with them. This action stops mounting debts from being passed on to a debt collector. Where your debt has already been passed to a debt collector then the best thing to do is to enter into a payment plan with them. You should be honest about any other debts you have, and be realistic about your capacity to pay the debt back.

Be very wary of companies promising to help you get out of debt or to consolidate it. They do not do this free and they may not even be able to do what they say they will. It is much better to access a financial counsellor connected to the government services. This service is free in Australia.

See the *Money Smart* website for more information on how to deal with debt collectors[112]. Information is also on the *Money Smart* website on financial counselling, debt consolidation, and refinancing, among other useful topics. There is a link discussing free legal advice, which is recommended at the point of contact from a debt collector, and also when there is a court proceeding against you.

SCAMS

It might be a good idea to arm yourself with some information about scams, so that you will be more likely to recognise one, and therefore avoid becoming a victim.

Read about companies you should not deal with, such as companies that are unlicensed, the tricks used, and how to protect yourself, at the *Money Smart* scam page[113].

One policy that can help to reduce any impulsivity in clicking on links or being sucked in is to say to yourself, 'nothing needs to be acted on immediately'.

If it's someone ringing up and claiming they are from some government agency or well-known company, the best thing to do is to tell them that you will ring that company yourself to confirm, and then just hang up.

Whether it's by text, over social media or by email, nothing needs acting on immediately. Sit back and think.

Go to the government website, *Scam Watch*[114] and see if there is anything similar to your experience there.

Also be cautious with unknown numbers on your mobile. Screening your calls is good for safety. If chatting with anyone on social media that you do not know in real life, you cannot be sure that they are who they say they are. One way you can get a bit of an idea is to check their profile page and look at the number of posts and how many friends or followers they have. If it's patchy, then don't respond. If they are flattering to you, they are much more likely to be scamming you. If they ask for money or for your personal details, it is definitely a scam.

SUMMARY

- Keep a record of income and expenses, so that you can work out your average spending. Keep track of everything you are spending.

- Work out your needs and wants, and look at reducing the number of things in the "wants" column.

- See if you can save up for an emergency fund.

- Stay away from payday loans, and avoid having more than one "buy now pay later" option at any one time, if at all possible.

- Look to ethical microfinance companies if you need some money to pay for an emergency, such as a broken fridge or washing machine.

- Contribute to your superannuation, and have income protection insurance and trauma cover, if you are employed.

- Increase your savings by choosing more economical options for socialising, reducing your clothing and lifestyle costs, buying food on special, and choosing to cook meals at home.

- Save up the deposit for your first home by remaining in the family home, if possible.

- By taking these steps, you can start being financially responsible and improve your money management.

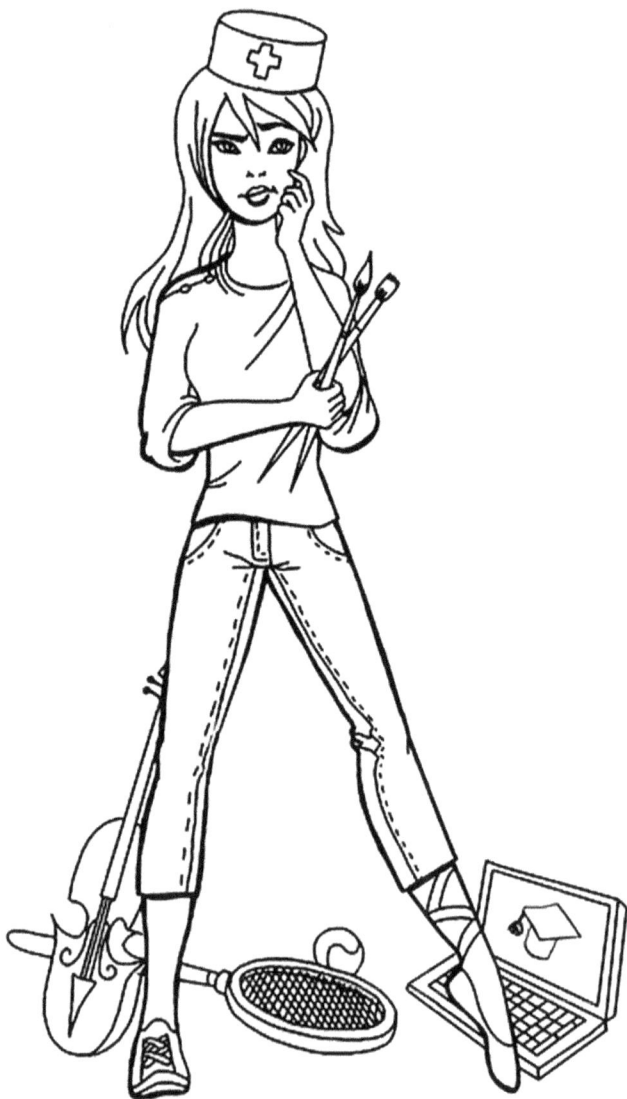

CHAPTER 8

WORK/CAREER

Do you approach change with flexibility and creativity?

We often define ourselves by our work. Our self-esteem can be tied up in this, so if we are not employed then our self-esteem takes a hit. If you are not employed, and it is not your choice, then you need to stay motivated to find work, or to find other ways to feel engaged with the world around you. Perhaps your situation means that at this point in time it isn't possible to find work. In this case, engagement with others may be helpful to provide social support and meaning.

DECIDING WHAT TO DO

You may make educational choices that are in line with your interests or talents, and you may finish school with the highest possible grades.

Whether you go on to university, attend a Technical and Further Education college (TAFE) or work towards an apprenticeship will depend on what you want to be and do.

Nowadays, you cannot bank on having a job for life. It is expected that the generations now coming into the workforce will have multiple jobs or careers throughout their lives. When setting out on a career path, if you go towards something that already interests you, whether that is academic, being around animals, or working with your hands, then you are more likely to find something you enjoy doing.

In this way, it might be possible to keep the number of career changes down to a minimum.

Changes may come where you try one area and find after a while that it doesn't work for you. Then you can carry it forward with you, see it as a learning experience and find something else. No learning is ever wasted. Professions with a high level of transferable skills are always going to be most helpful in this regard.

Where you don't do as well as you hoped or expected in high school or university, then all is not lost. It is not the case that your life depends on your exam results—at any stage whatsoever. You could consider a gap year, and during this time investigate certain areas you are interested in. Perhaps gain some work experience and follow your interests.

Even if you do not get the best results, you can still go to university if that is what you want to do. There are multiple pathways to university, and if you choose to wait to enrol, there is always mature age entry, which is around twenty-five years of age.

Even if you failed Year 12, you are able to do a qualifying year of study that means you can start your preferred course degree on completion. University is by no means the province of 19–20-year-olds. Whether you pass Year 12 or not, you can go to university at any age. It can even be a better experience if you leave it until you are a little older, when you may be more certain that the degree you want to complete is the right one for you.

Alternatively, you might consider going into a trade, where you learn on the job, along with some technical education. You might consider plumbing, electricals, or mechanics. In Australia, these types of technical courses are run by TAFE colleges. Make an appointment with one of the course advisers for a run down on what the course entails, and have a discussion around making your choices.

Where you don't want to embark on a trade or go to university then do your research around other training options. Explore what is available through private institutions. There are many options, and if you can settle on something you are interested in then you are on your way.

While your parents may be encouraging you to go into a particular career, you should really look at what that career involves and work out whether your personality traits and your talents are suited to that path.

The question you can ask yourself is, 'Would I enjoy doing that?'

It might be helpful to talk to a careers adviser and find out more about the tasks that are involved. Are those tasks activities that you can see yourself doing? Not all tasks in all jobs are necessarily fun. However, if you can see yourself being ok about doing them then that is one hurdle you will be able to jump.

It is important to be able to see yourself enjoying the majority of the tasks, or at least to enjoy the result of engaging in those tasks. There must be an emotional payoff for you. Whether it is getting satisfaction from helping people, or creating something that you are proud of, you should be able to envisage or imagine positive outcomes.

ASSESSING YOURSELF

Think about careers that might utilise your interests, talents and the subjects you are good at.

Get careers advice. Talk to people. You can also do a careers interest survey, which was originally created by Holland[115] and is available free online[116]. You can then look at the jobs that are involved in your interest profile.

Holland splits up careers into six areas. They are: realistic, artistic, investigative, social, enterprising, and conventional. Find your top three areas. Then you can think about which jobs you might like. This is only a first step, and you could investigate these possibilities further with a career's adviser or other professional. It also allows you to select and explore jobs in particular categories and at different education levels. If anything interests you, then you can take steps to find out more.

FUTURE PROSPECTS

Over time due to technology changes and societal change, employment and jobs tend to shift around and while some kinds of work appear, others disappear. No matter the time when you are planning or looking actively for employment the one constant area of need will be in human services and care, and in jobs that have interpersonal interactions at their core.

Jobs involving communication and interpersonal skills are likely to be preserved, and even to increase in their importance[117]. Consider these areas in your assessment of your work prospects and interests.

At any stage of your life, you can create change, you can find different areas to work in or careers to transition to. With increasing environmental and climate pressures, many people will be required to help the transition to a cleaner and more sustainable future.

Explore aspects around where your interests lie. People skills, technological skills, and logistical skills will be really needed so that we can get everything up and running smoothly.

We will need people trained in all the natural sciences so that we can monitor, and engage in, saving ourselves and the natural world—and perhaps the economy and all that goes with it too. Such a wide range to choose from!

There may also be great opportunities to create your own career, where you are providing services, logistics, and information in any area that impacts peoples' lives. Fields such as engineering and the sciences would be included here.

Additionally, providing services to help underprivileged sections of society and making their lives better is an admirable career goal. As would bringing more awareness to any aspect of climate change and our need for sustainable and practical solutions, so that we can begin to reduce our carbon output in real terms. In is a fact that Australia is one of the heaviest carbon emitters per capita in the world at the time of writing[118].

Sometimes it is difficult to really know what you want to do before you have had some life experience. There are some advantages to knowing what you want to do early on. However, for many people who change careers, having experience in a different field can also be of great benefit, as you will be bringing something outside the norm to your new career, which can give you an edge.

WORK EXPERIENCE

Trying out a role before you take on a full-time job provides you with some insight into what the role entails. Work experience can help you to sort out what you want to do, or at least, what you don't want to do.

Working front of house in a café or fast-food outlet when you are young can stand you in good stead when you're older, as employers are always after people with customer-facing experience. It's always helpful to be able to carry out a number of jobs, as having a wide range of skills gives you a stronger platform from which to find more work, if and when you need to.

It may be that you are looking for work, but have not yet been able to find anywhere to take you on. It is tough when you are just starting out, as you may have the right qualifications but you don't have the experience.

If you're finding it difficult to land a job, it is important not to give up. Try further afield, where it is practical for you to do so. In this process, consider going further in terms of distance where possible. Another option could be to consider your transferable skills and begin to apply for positions that are more your second or third preference, instead of your first preference. You can also try different industries, sectors or size of business, including government or corporate occupations.

TAKING UP OPPORTUNITIES

John's grandfather took him aside one day. He told him that when it came to employment, to always say 'yes' when someone asked him to do something. John asked, 'What if I can't do it?' His Grandfather replied, 'You still say yes, and then you go out and learn how to do it.'

Saying 'yes' means taking opportunities as they arise, as well as expanding your skill set. This opens up new pathways for you in life. It is worth noting that saying 'yes' to new challenges is different to not being able to say 'no' if it is something you really don't want to do or genuinely won't be able to learn in a timely fashion—you still need to set boundaries and be realistic.

EXPLORATION

When looking for work or changing employment, it is best to check advertisements in all areas: online and offline, as well as canvassing firms and businesses directly.

There are some jobs that you may get through being head hunted or through your social networks, such as *LinkedIn*. Make sure you have an updated

Curriculum Vitae or resume to send to prospective employers. It is also required to have a cover letter for the specific job you are applying for. Handing in a first-class application is crucial particularly for some jobs. You may find help online, or from a professional CV writer to enhance your professional application.

INTERVIEWS

In any interview, appearance and presentation is important. Dress as formally as the position warrants. It is better to be slightly overdressed than to be too casual.

Good hygiene is a must. It may be helpful to think about the questions you might be asked in an interview, and to work out some good answers.

You might know a business manager or someone who may be able to do a mock interview with you. It is common to be nervous in a job interview. The more practice you get the less nervous you will be, and the better the outcome.

In exploring advertisements to apply for, it sometimes helps to be adventurous.

JOSH'S STORY

Josh came across an advertisement for a copywriter. This was what he was interested in doing for a career. He was not sure that he had the experience and ability to get the job, but after thinking about it for a while he said to himself, *what have I got to lose?* He applied for the position, and although he didn't have much experience, he gave thoughtful answers in his interview and was able to present a great portfolio of ideas he had created as examples of his work, even though they were only for imaginary companies. His engagement and initiative landed him the job.

The moral of this story is to go for jobs that you think you might not get, regardless of your uncertainty of the outcome. This holds for anyone. You need to have confidence in your ability to work in a position that might be a little out of your comfort zone. All jobs are initially unknown, and it is perfectly normal to feel anxious and uncertain to start with. Just diving in might well be the right way to do it.

WORK RELATIONSHIPS

Where you have managed to land a job, then you need to pay attention to your work relationships.

Respect everyone, and treat them in the way you would like to be treated. If you prefer to keep some distance and just have minimum contact then this is your choice; you don't need to tell your co-workers your life story, but at least be friendly.

Give yourself a couple of months to find out the culture and systems of communication that are in place. You can then choose how much you want to involve yourself with everyone at work.

The culture of a work place is more than the stated rules; it also includes the unspoken rules that exist in any group.

Each company or business has a culture, and it may take a little while for you to figure out the dynamics and expectations. Everyone may work hard during the week but go to the pub on Friday nights, for instance. You can decide whether you want to socialise with your work mates or not. In a general sense, where you are able to remain pleasant and assertive with your colleagues, then you will maintain your independence. If you do become close friends with some people, then you may need to think about how this may impact on impartiality and neutrality, and what steps you can take to ensure you maintain both your integrity and your friendships. You don't want to find yourself in a situation where you are asked to "take sides", as this could cause problems either personally or professionally. While this may not be an issue it is something to consider, so that you can be prepared in the event that conflict does arise.

Work relationships can be easy or difficult, depending on personalities and status. If you are starting out at entry level, you may have a number of managers above you. At work, respect is the best value to show. This is not to say that you can't stand up for yourself. It is important to stand up for yourself if others are taking advantage of you. Knowing how to be assertive is helpful. You can set boundaries for yourself and others, and there is a right way of going about this. Assertiveness is not being aggressive, but it is looking after your needs and respecting the needs of others.

HOW TO SUCCEED IN THE WORKPLACE

Work is a serious business, so fooling around and practical jokes are generally a bad idea. However, that doesn't mean you can't have a laugh about something, bearing in mind that laughing with others about something is very different from laughing at someone.

Respectful conversation and behaviour are called for. Being polite and helping when asked are behaviours that will be rewarded by more positive relationships.

If you want to have a good reputation amongst your colleagues then it is better to be on your best behaviour at all times, even at office parties or team-building events.

Getting drunk, behaving stupidly or pairing off with a work colleague are not things that will help your reputation. Behave in ways that will show you are responsible, honest, reliable, and dependable. If you say you'll do something, then do it. If you maintain positive relationships with everyone possible then you will be in a stronger position if and when the time comes for you to step up to a more responsible role. Remember, actions affect your reputation as well, and it's always better to under-promise and over-deliver, than giving a promise and failing to fulfill it.

WHEN TROUBLE COMES

When an issue arises with a co-worker, whether a major disagreement or a minor disagreement, then it is better to sort it out with them straight away. It is counterproductive to discuss the situation with other co-workers before you approach the person concerned. If you try to sort it out through being assertive, but after a couple of attempts it still doesn't get sorted, then you could approach your boss, manager, or the Human Resource department or person if there is one. They should be able to help. If your manager is not responsive, you may wish to take things to a higher level. See the chapter on assertiveness for more information.

In a situation where you are being bullied by someone at work, then even if you are assertive, it may be completely disregarded. It would be a good idea to analyse what is happening and talk to someone outside of work about it.

If it is a co-worker bullying you then you can talk to your boss about it. If it's your boss, then your organisation should have a policy about workplace bullying and you could take your complaint to Human Resources or a specific person within the organisation.

If there is a Human Resources department, there may be an opportunity for free counselling through the Employee Assistance Program. If you cannot get the help you require within your workplace, you may need to seek help from an official government body. There are national anti-bullying laws and state or territory health and safety bodies that can help people with bullying and harassment in the workplace.

The *Fair Work Ombudsman* should be the first point of contact to ensure your rights are being protected and upheld[119]. On the *Fair Work* website, there are also help pages that give guidance on work conditions, including pay[120].

POSITIVE FEELINGS

Where everyone relates well with the others in a workplace then you will be more likely to feel good about going to work. If it is usually a happy place then the feelings generated are more positive than when conflict frequently arises.

RACHEL'S STORY

Rachel has learnt to surround herself with people who make her happy. When she started out as a hairdresser, she wasn't happy and was always being put down by the other hairdressers in the salon where she worked. She felt as though she was worthless and could never grow or become anything. When she lost her job at the salon, she became so shut down that she didn't even want to be a hairdresser anymore. However, after a while she found a new job at a salon where she was much happier. It took a while to find her confidence again, but it gradually happened. If she had known how different her experiences of work life could be, she would have left her old job much sooner to become happier and be the best she could be.

> Rachel learned that having a good professional life requires surrounding yourself with people who make you feel it's worth waking up and going to work.

Another situation that is not uncommon in the workplace is sexual attraction.

It could be helpful to consider the ramifications before you jump into a relationship. Issues to think about include workplace rules about such liaisons, and the possible consequences if the relationship doesn't work out. Would you feel comfortable continuing to work with, and possibly also socialise with, your former partner?

If your current employment is in an environment that you love and is providing you with great career opportunities, then explore what being in a relationship with someone who shares that environment with you could mean. Consider all aspects and talk about it with your prospective partner before diving in.

It isn't that work relationships are not advisable, but rather that in some circumstances and in some organisations, they are not conducive to promotion or positive outcomes in the long run. In some organisations there are rules against relationships among employees.

BEING YOUR BEST

The best position to be in at work is to fit in, but also maintain an element of independence. Doing a good job and upholding the rules of behaviour laid down by your workplace will mean that you are welcomed and valued as an employee.

You can make up your own mind about what to share about yourself and what to keep to yourself. At least initially, it is best to err on the side of caution and only share what you need to in order to carry out your job to the best of your ability. Essentially, your behaviour at work will actually give others some idea of who you are as a person. The more you can carry out your job in a pleasant and ordered way, the better the impression you will give. Thus, the better you will be thought of as an employee. Additionally, if you show respect to everyone you work with, are honest, and are able to be assertive, then you will be standing up for yourself and others, and feeling capable and empowered.

Once you are settled and happy in your place of work, you may have the opportunity to rise up the ranks. Such opportunities will depend on the organisation and the hierarchical structure of the positions within it. The higher you go, the more responsibilities you will have in relation to your work load, your employer, and any colleagues you are managing. This also holds true if you are in business for yourself and engage employees to work for you.

Managing is an important role, and being a leader requires emotional intelligence and people skills. It is, however, a role that can be learned and practised, so there is hope if you are not a natural leader.

In any kind of work and employment, it can be helpful if you find what you are doing is meaningful and purposeful in some way. There are many different jobs and positions available, from unskilled menial jobs that need to be done by someone, through to complex jobs that require in depth knowledge and specialist skills.

Regardless of your position, how you perceive the value of your work is, to a very great extent, what will help you to find meaning in whatever you are doing.

This is purpose. Having a sense of purpose in your life is what helps you have better mental health and better overall wellbeing, including lower mortality[121] than if you hate what you are doing or otherwise find no satisfaction in it. The good news is that you can improve your perception of purpose by exploring the greater object or aim that your work may provide for others. A purpose isn't purely about making money. A good purpose would be to help others, to be of service to others in some way in order to make their lives better. If you can think about your purpose in this way, then even if the job itself is very menial, boring, or whatever, then you may find more meaning in the role.

SUMMARY

- Choose a career that falls within your sphere of interests and skills.

- Ensure your talents and personality are in sync.

- Make sure work relationships are built around respect.

- Choose how little or how much you associate with people at work.

- Be assertive and stand up for yourself if you feel you are being expected to do too much.

- Seek help and support if you are being bullied. Carry out your work in a pleasant and efficient manner, and treat clients, employers, and co-workers with respect, in order to be recognised as a valued employee.

- Take calculated risks to help you to advance your career and ensure you continue to learn and grow.

- Find a sense of purpose, whether you are already doing something that you love or not.

- It's ok to switch jobs and careers but it's helpful to have a plan B to fall back on while you are transitioning.

- By taking these steps, you can begin to build a career of your dreams.

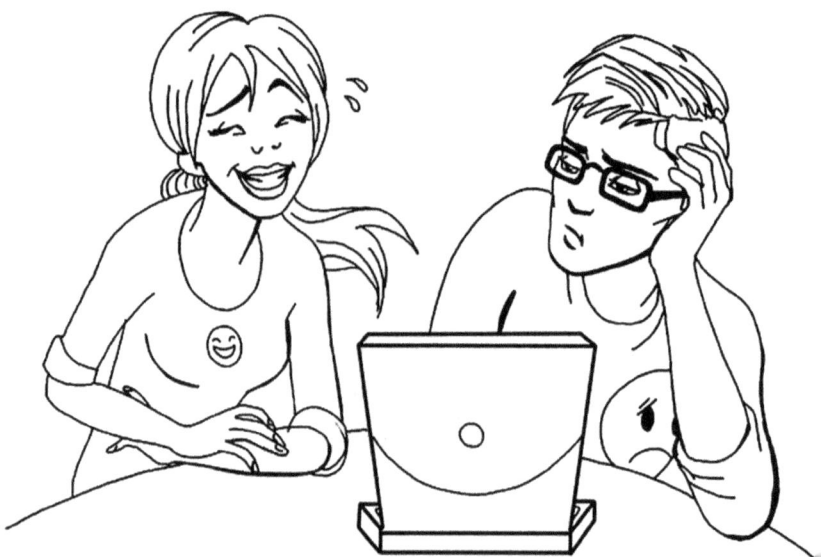

CHAPTER 9

EMOTIONAL LIFE

Are you in charge of your emotions or are your emotions in charge of you?

We are emotional beings. We experience emotions in numerous ways. We make value judgements using emotion, such as choosing one product over another, because we prefer the packaging or because we liked the advertisement.

A value judgement occurs when we decide that one thing is better than another. We feel emotions that are attached to events in our memories, and we feel emotions as we experience situations throughout the day. The way in which making value judgements utilises the emotions is shown in those people who have an isolated and specific brain injury to the central (or ventromedial) portion of the frontal lobes. This is the part of the brain that processes emotion. What may happen is that they find it impossible to choose one thing over another, when there is not much difference between them, except perhaps, ordinarily one may be favoured over the other[122]. Even in trivial choices, we use emotion.

As previously discussed, genetics and our early environment play a part in how we respond to situations, events, and circumstances. How we have come to respond and react to certain internal and external events is essentially a habit. Just because we have responded in one way all our life so far, doesn't mean that it is forever. We can change. We can recreate new pathways in our brains because of neuroplasticity (which is the brain's capacity to continue to evolve and grow from life experience). What this means is that if you are suffering from emotional issues, you have the capacity to change your brain. This means that if you often feel particular emotions, such as shame or guilt, it doesn't have to be permanent[123].

Epigenetics shows that through changing your internal environment, including your perspectives and beliefs, you are able to turn specific genes in your DNA off or on. Whether you are affecting specific genes or whether you are creating smaller changes in your brain such as programming your neurons to fire along different pathways that lead to better outcomes for you, to some extent does not matter. What does matter is that you are able to make these changes through discovering the right ways of thinking and feeling for you. In this way, you can change your experience and life. What this ultimately means is that you are *not* doomed to continue to live in the same space in your mind *if you don't want to.*

THE LOWDOWN ON EMOTION

When talking about emotion, it is very helpful to use the right word in labelling the emotion. There are many words that describe emotions. A list that may be reasonably comprehensive can be found at www.dianahutchison.com/shop and you are welcome to download it so that you can refer to it when you wish.

By using the right word when talking to another person about how you feel, or what you felt, you will convey an accurate picture of what you are experiencing or have experienced. Communication then improves. The more accurate you can be with your descriptions of how you feel, the more others will understand you. If you say you feel bad, this does not convey a specific picture, whereas saying you feel guilty conveys a lot more to the listener and they will be able to understand your experience better.

In remembering events, we can easily recall the emotion we were feeling at the time. The more intense the emotion, the greater likelihood of us remembering the event. Once we are feeling a particular emotion then it seems as though there is a pathway in our brains that connects all the events that are attached to that particular emotion, which means they are much easier to access.

So, emotions are attached to events or situations. Thoughts and feelings are also connected. Emotions guide our thoughts—although there is also an element of interpreting the situation you find yourself in. Many factors are involved in this process, not least of which is the mind/body connection and the ability of your body/intuition to alert you to a threat.

Thoughts and feelings are inextricably linked. If you are feeling unhappy, and you consciously think more happy thoughts and remember times when you were happy, then your mood often changes. This is likely to help in everyday situations, but may not work as well if you are particularly depressed. See the chapters on mental health and personal growth for further information on this issue.

In everyday situations, though, if you choose and are motivated to do so, you have the capacity and opportunity to change how you feel. It would help if you have a store of positive memories to call upon.

In recognising and labelling emotions, we gain self-awareness in the present moment. The more we do this, the more we can increase our self-awareness. We can quite easily accept normal emotions. It's when we feel extremes of emotion, and particularly negative emotions, that we may need to take some action for ourselves.

You can't make others do or feel what you want them to: you can only change yourself. People don't necessarily see things in the way you do. Everyone has different histories, values, beliefs, and ways of thinking. Emotions arise due to past experiences and thoughts, and your own set of experiences lead to the view you have of your world. It is possible to rise above this.

You can do this by using empathy. That is, by putting yourself into someone else's shoes. Empathy is not sympathy. You are not going into your own emotions when you empathise. It is more about the understanding of where the other person is. It is taking the framework of the other person's story and putting yourself in that story, in order to understand how and why that person is feeling the way they are. You show empathy when you are actively listening to the other person and reflecting back in their own words what they are feeling. Sometimes just listening really helps someone to express how they are feeling and this by itself is beneficial. A situation can be discussed and sometimes, at a later date, options may be explored, and solutions found and actioned. While it depends on what the situation is, your emotional reaction will be uniquely yours. This is due to your worldview, past experiences, and the meaning you place on whatever is happening.

SELF-MONITORING

In order to create even small changes within ourselves, it is helpful to be able to get out of the subjective or personal point of view or perspective. The subjective perspective is, of course, you seeing things from exactly your point of view. Where you want to get to is the observer perspective where you are looking at a situation from outside of that situation you are in. From this perspective it is easier to be more logical, objective and realistic about what is happening in a communication situation with others.

Thus, in the subjective or personal perspective we are aware of ourselves and what we are saying, thinking, feeling, and behaving. In order to know what to change and how, getting into the observer role so that you can put self-monitoring into place is important. You are going from being aware in the personal perspective, and being in you, to being in the observer role where you are objectively seeing what is happening so that can then start to monitor yourself. Self-monitoring means you are taking that step back from awareness, so you are aware of being aware.

As you go through your day take note of what happens. You may like to flag particular situations so you can start self-monitoring when these situations arise. Take note of the sequence of events and behaviours, what you said and what the other person said, what you felt, and what the end result was. This is the start. Now you have a baseline to work from and will be able to put new behaviours into place on the next occasion. For more information and details on this see my previous book, *A Practical Guide for Self Change.*

If you are in an unhealthy relationship, how do you recognise it? You may recognise that it is an unhealthy relationship when you realise that you feel more negative emotions when you are with the person, or when you are away from this person but thinking about them. If you feel sad because of what they do; if they say things that make you feel worthless, helpless, and hopeless; if they criticise you and put you down all the time; if they take advantage of you and you feel downtrodden, these are all signs that either the relationship itself needs to change in some way or perhaps that you need to get out of it.

Where you approach your partner and ask for change but they refuse to engage in any relationship counselling or refuse to change their behaviour, then it may be time to seek individual counselling to change yourself and find support to remove yourself from that relationship. Revisit Chapters 4 and 5 for more focus on this.

HAPPINESS

Happiness is a state of mind in the present, not an end result. People say that they will be happy when they achieve a certain outcome, whether it's a job, a partner, or something that is in the future.

However, why wait to be happy when you can be happy as you move towards these goals? You don't need to wait to be happy. All that needs to be happening for you is that you have some positive things to be grateful for. Then you can say to yourself, '*I am healthy, I am grateful for my health, I am grateful for my friends, I am grateful that I am progressing towards my goals.*'

Allow yourself to be happy for forward movement. Happiness is an uplifting of your spirit. It is also good for your immune system. Perhaps we are not going to feel happy every minute of the day, but you can feel happy most of the time. And then you can say that you are happy. Don't discount feelings of happiness just because you feel upset about something for a time. The positive feelings you have need to be taken into account. If you see yourself as making progress and you have a number of things to be grateful for, then you can feel positively about your situation and can feel happy.

The more positive statements you can say to yourself about where you are at, the happier you will feel. Give yourself the benefit of the doubt and give yourself the chance to feel happy. You will find that everything looks better when you are feeling more balanced, and then it is possible to spiral up rather than down. In the morning, or last thing at night, find at least three things that you are grateful for, and say them to yourself. Grateful people are usually happier people.

ANGER

All emotions are legitimate. Everyone feels anger at one time or another. The question is how you express your anger and whether you act in ways that have negative consequences for yourself and/ or others. Just being shouted at can have negative consequences, let alone being the victim of violence.

In nearly all circumstances violence is not the answer. The only time it is warranted is in self-defence against a physical attack. Otherwise, words are a better way to deal with a situation that makes you angry. Talking things through and using reasoning and logic is much more helpful.

One strategy to manage your anger is to take yourself out of the situation for a time so that you can calm down. Then, once you are calm, talk things through sensibly. Another strategy is to count to ten before you reply. Taking a few moments to compose yourself can sometimes be enough to take the edge off and allow you to reply more calmly.

Becoming aggressive is not the way to resolve a situation. It will almost certainly just make it worse. It is better to be assertive. In being assertive, you state your needs in the situation and stand up for yourself. In addition, you take other person's needs into account. Where you are assertive rather than aggressive or passive, then you are more likely to feel better about your behaviour, better about yourself, and better about the situation. When you address situations as they arise then you are less likely to explode with anger at a later date. You are able to state how you feel, and this allows some expression of your emotion, which in turn reduces the likelihood of bottling things up. See the chapter on assertiveness for more information.

Overall, statistics show that men are more violent towards women than the other way around[124]. This may come down to societal values and norms. Just because this happens does not make it ok. Men need to change how they deal with anger and change how they think about women. Women are not property or objects. Men and women are equal partners in a relationship, and women need to be treated as such by all men.

DIFFICULT EMOTIONS

We will look at strategies to manage the more difficult emotions now.

Difficult emotions, such as sadness and loneliness, can arise because we are thinking thoughts that bring these emotions up for us. Every emotion is normal and within the realm of human experience. All emotions are legitimate.

Generally speaking, unless you consciously think about negative emotions and keep playing them over and over in your mind (called rumination), emotions will only last a certain amount of time. However, if you consciously go with them and think about all the times you felt that particular emotion, then you will feel that emotion for longer. If you don't feed it, you won't have it staying around. This is because your emotions are fed by your thoughts. If you think different thoughts, then your emotions will change. There is a difference between dwelling on negative feelings and being aware of your emotions. By being aware, and focusing on what you are feeling, then the emotion may change by itself. This is the idea behind the book *Focussing* by Gendlin[125]. Each time the emotion changes, you label it, and then keep on focusing on what you are feeling. Then it changes again.

Although different emotions are fed by our thoughts, we may have particular issues to which negative emotions are attached. In this case, we will continue to feel the negative emotions whenever we are reminded of the issue or are triggered by an internal or external thought or situation that brings it all back to our mind. This will continue to happen until the event or issue has been processed more completely and the emotion is detached from the event or issue, or has otherwise been resolved. Processing the event or issue through counselling, psychotherapy or other emotional processing strategies is the best way to reduce the emotions attached to the event or issue. NLP and Time Line Therapy™ are two other modalities for processing past events and issues you may have.

STRATEGIES TO MANAGE FEELINGS

There are different strategies to manage different emotions. Because people may feel the same emotion for different reasons, each person needs to find the action that works for them. If you feel sad, and if this is because you have experienced a loss of some kind, then it may be helpful to experience that sadness for a while, label it, explore the reason, and then focus on what you are doing. If you are feeling sad because of someone's actions or behaviour towards you, then acknowledge this to yourself, think about how you could act to redress this feeling, and work out what you can say in an assertive manner to the person responsible to try and change the situation. Sometimes action may be appropriate, and sometimes it won't be helpful. Sometimes, if you just focus on the feeling then the feeling may change to a different emotion. However, you need to give yourself time to actually feel the emotion in order to progress.

A strategy for managing the feeling of loneliness may be to take action to contact the outside world. This may be possible if you have someone to phone, whether a friend or a counselling service. The feeling of loneliness may go away after contact. Where you feel lonely but are in the midst of many people, then this may indicate the need for individual counselling to contact the inner you. Going out with friends, seeing family or phoning them, or even going out people watching may be helpful strategies to reduce loneliness. Talking to random strangers, such as the cashier at the supermarket checkout, can also be a way to feel more connected to the world and less lonely[126],[127].

Envy and jealousy are emotions that are quite unnecessary. What is the use of feeling that someone else has it better than you? You have your life and they have theirs. The strategy to dealing with these emotions is to consider yourself and your world as giving you the best at the current time. It is much better to be happy for others who have a good life, or who are in a better position than you. If you can be happy for them, then you are not condemning yourself to being in the same position forever. If you can be happy for others then you are giving yourself the opportunity to change to a better situation. Focusing on positive feelings is much better than focusing on negative feelings. What we focus on grows. Where you focus on lack, lack grows. Where you focus on abundance, abundance grows. Focus on positive things and emotions so that you will be able to notice opportunities to change your situation for the better.

FORGIVENESS AND OTHER EMOTIONS

If someone has hurt you in some way, no matter whether the situation is big or small, you may have many different complex emotions to deal with afterwards. I am only discussing the emotions here, not the external or physical aspects. Where these are present, then obviously they need attending to.

So, where you feel emotionally hurt, other emotions may arise. These may include anger, resentment, revenge and other possibly what might be called negative emotions. It is completely normal to feel a range of emotions when we feel, for instance, that others have invaded or upset our boundaries and sense of self.

As previously discussed, you cannot change someone else's behaviour or internal thinking process. You can only change yourself.

It is the case that what you may be thinking or believing, is not actually affecting the other person(s). Whether you are stewing over a situation, ruminating and staying in the negative emotions of hurt, anger, revenge and so on, is not having one iota of difference or any effect on them. Essentially, you are only hurting yourself.

What these emotions do is to create in your body the right environment to create more stress and that may have an effect on *you* - of possibly chronic stress which, as already discussed can lead to health issues. Additionally, if you remain stuck in those negative emotions, it may impede your ability to feel happy, lighter and your capacity to move forward in life.

The best thing you can do is to let go of your feelings towards the other person through forgiving them. This is not to say that you need to tell them you forgive them. This forgiveness is an inner process that you do for *yourself*, so that the emotions don't fester inside you and harm you.

You have the choice when you do this. If you have experienced deep trauma, it may not be the right time yet. Self-forgiveness heals our unconscious mind and allows healing to take place at a deep level. This forgiveness exercise also seems to have a tangible effect on how you relate with others, as well as how you see yourself in relation to the person or people involved. You are likely to feel freer and lighter.

FORGIVENESS EXERCISE

Imagine the person standing in front of you, surrounded in pink light. Say out loud to them, 'I ask your forgiveness, I forgive you, I forgive myself. I pray for your prospering, wherever you are. I bless you and release you to your highest good'.

This process will dissolve the emotions and allow you to move forward with your life.

You can also use this exercise if you have guilty feelings about something you've done.

Resentment and frustration can be problematic feelings to overcome. Resentments usually build up over time. Sometimes they are prevalent within a primary relationship. Whenever an argument occurs, all the resentments come up and out to be raked over again.

Again, you can try using the forgiveness exercise and see if the resentments dissolve. At other times, proper discussion and feeling heard is an important road to peace, for both parties. The same can be said about frustration. Something is not happening the way you want it to. Sometimes rational discussion and asking for behaviour change can be helpful. Relationship counselling may also be beneficial.

PROCESSING NEGATIVE EMOTIONS

Where you experience inappropriate amounts of negative emotions you may find Time Line Therapy™ helpful. This is a creative imagination process that is a way of processing past events, and attached emotions that can be conscious or unconscious and allowing new perspectives to occur that contribute to healing. While this process does not mean that you won't feel the negative emotion again, it is usual for the edge to be taken off, so that the excessive degree of the emotion dissolves.

Time Line Therapy™ can be provided by an NLP Practitioner who has trained in this area, and can be pursued alone or in conjunction with other NLP therapy or, depending on the practitioner, when working on your issues with the aim of self-change.

Meditation and mindfulness can also be useful in reducing the amount of reactivity you feel on a daily basis. Counselling, including psychological counselling and psychotherapy are also beneficial. If you can find someone to teach you the Emotional Freedom Technique (EFT) then you can practice this yourself, which would help you to become more in control of your emotions.

WHEN UNDERSTANDING OTHERS' EMOTIONS IS DIFFICULT

Sometimes it is difficult to understand what others may be experiencing, feeling, or what their idea of the world is. We all have an idea of how our mind works, and how the world works. As we get older, we refine these ideas until hopefully we have a good working model in our minds that works at least most of the time. We actually keep on refining this throughout our lives based on many factors including our experiences and beliefs.

If you do find it difficult to understand others, and that person or person(s) are part of a group that are different from you, there are some actions you can take to gain more understanding. One option is to ask them to tell you their story of their experiences. Obviously, where the situation is appropriate for this to happen, this is an option. Another option is for you to discover more about their general situation where this is possible. Since we all have the same needs and wants, through hearing or understanding their stories better and finding out what happened for them to get to where they are, it will become easier to appreciate their lives. Everyone is worthy of respect and love.

Where you find some difficulties with various individuals, and it becomes an issue for you, then consider having counselling to help you find out more about yourself and how you interact with others. This may be of benefit in the long term.

SUMMARY

- Understand that all emotions are legitimate and a part of our lives.

- Learn to recognise that thoughts and emotions are linked.

- Work towards living in the present moment and being grateful for what and who you have in your life, in order to increase more positive emotions of happiness, joy, and love.

- Explore the different ways that negative emotions can be processed, to release them from past events.

- Consider mindfulness or counselling, if you are feeling overwhelmed by negative thoughts and emotions.

- Allow yourself to feel your emotions, and understand that this is part of the process of letting go.

- If you can accept your emotions, and not allow them to control your behaviour in negative ways, then you are gaining authenticity.

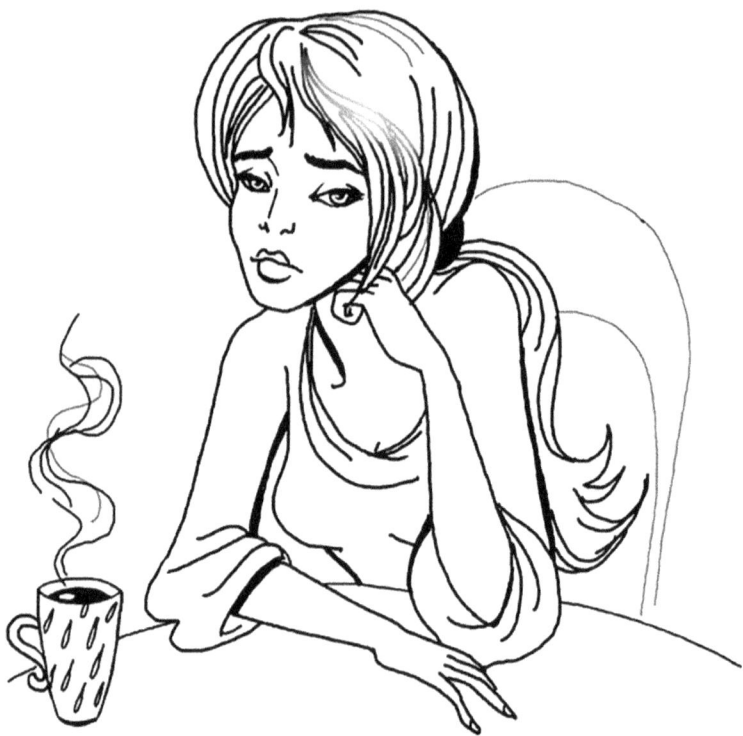

CHAPTER 10

MENTAL HEALTH

How do you define mental health in relation to your own life, and in relation to other people's lives? Are these definitions different?

WHAT IS MENTAL HEALTH?

Mental health includes our emotional, psychological, and social well-being. It affects how we think, feel, and act. Additionally, it helps determine how we handle stress, relate to others, and make healthy choices[128]. Mental health is important all through life.

When you are mentally healthy you have a clear mind, you are able to focus on what you are doing, you are acting in the world without fear and making progress towards your goals. There is nothing specifically that is bothering you, apart from the normal day-to-day challenges, you communicate reasonably well, and feel that you are an agent of change in your life. Although you may not be perfect and could possibly make some changes, you are essentially an effective human being. Your emotions are generally neutral to positive, and you are usually able to let go of negative thoughts.

When mental health issues arise, these things may change, and your way of being in the world may be impacted. Examples of this include:

- You usually have a clear mind and it starts to get less clear

- You are no longer able to focus on what you used to focus on, as a result of competing thoughts and emotions.

- You find you are fearful of something specific happening to you or your loved ones.

- You suddenly change your goals to something others would not agree with.

- You find specific issues or things start to bother you a lot and interfere with your daily life.

- Your emotional life changes to very negative or very positive but destructive.

- You dwell on very negative thoughts and are unable to think positively.

While these are some things to watch out for, even if you find yourself experiencing some or all of these changes, you are not alone. It's helpful to get a professional opinion and to seek appropriate treatment where applicable. About 44% of people experience mental illness in the course of their lifetime, so it is very common. If you encounter such a challenge, you are not alone. Around 2 in 5 people in Australia experience mental health issues over their lifetime[129].

Mental health problems are not something others can see, or maybe even notice, unless your behaviour changes or you tell someone. If someone knows you well, then they may ask what's wrong. But generally speaking, no one will know what you are experiencing just by looking at you.

If you start to feel different from how you usually feel, whether more anxious, more depressed, or whatever, a good policy is to tell your loved ones and discuss it. If you find you cannot manage the differences in the way you think or feel on your own, and that your thoughts or feelings are interfering with your daily life, then asking for help and reaching out is the best thing to do. Your mental health is important, and asking for help and getting it is far better than continuing to suffer alone.

Understanding both our own mental health and that of others enables us to be more proactive and insightful about what may be going on for other people. This means that using empathy, making choices for ourselves, asking how others are, and including them in making decisions about things that will have an impact on them, can be an addition to our conversations. We can consider how we may be affected by engaging in a particular activity, and how others may be too—not just physically, but emotionally and mentally.

There is still some stigma around mental illness, but not as much now as there used to be. There are a few points to consider generally:

- There are crisis phone lines to call. In Australia, these include Lifeline and Headspace.

- You can also approach family or friends if you need someone to talk to.

- It is important to find the right doctor, psychiatrist, or therapist for you. Shop around to find a person who is empathic and encouraging.

- Therapists, psychologists, and counsellors can only help you as much as you allow—you need to engage in your own healing process.

- Equally, therapists, psychologists, and counsellors can only help you as far as they themselves have gone—in understanding, experience, and personal growth.

- Explore what particular external factors could be having an effect, such as dietary, social, situational, lifestyle and other factors.

- It might be a good option, depending on your problem, to consider joining a program or group that is specifically for your age group that enables you to engage in an activity of some kind. This can help you make friends and feel less disconnected, which will likely improve how you are feeling.

DEPRESSION

We have discussed how thoughts and feelings/ emotions are connected, and how it is possible to change your mood.

Sometimes, the emotion is so powerful that trying to change it consciously is just too difficult. In this case, your brain chemicals may be having a powerful effect, so it may take longer to affect some change in the way you are feeling.

As previously discussed, a particular emotion allows access to memories of similar states and the thoughts that go with them. These feelings and thoughts can override conscious efforts to think of other things. However, it is still worth making the attempt. Thinking of possible positive outcomes and benefits that may help. There may be a positive in the situation that you are unable to see at the time.

Talking with someone may be helpful if this is the case. You can try your family and friends for a start.

If you are still feeling down, then find a counsellor or psychologist. Having counselling from a trained professional has been shown to be helpful in recovery from depression[130]. A counsellor can be a good sounding board, and can help you set some realistic and specific goals that you can take action towards. It may take some weeks, but you can change your thinking about your situation.

Exercise is also helpful for depression, as is engaging in activities that usually make you happy. You might be depressed due to an event in your life or because your life is not going in the way you really want. You may then see the light at the end of the tunnel.

Where you are clinically depressed, which is further down the road to feeling hopeless or helpless, then your medical doctor or general practitioner (GP) can refer you to a psychologist with a Mental Health Care Plan (in Australia).

Sometimes medication may be indicated, but make sure that you discuss the possible side effects with your doctor or your psychiatrist, if you are referred to one. Make an informed decision about whether to go on medication or not. Ensure that your doctor makes up a Mental Health Care Plan of six sessions and refers you to a psychologist.

For some people, it is very difficult to come off medication. There is a genetic component to depression, and what this means is that some people find certain medications help to some extent, but that they do not experience a full recovery from their symptoms.

Generally, with depression, you are stuck either in the past or in the future, rather than living in the moment. It is when we bring our awareness more into the present moment, allow the future to unfold, and release ourselves from our past, that we can find more vibrancy and meaning to our life right now.

It may be that you are able to recover with some lifestyle changes, such as diet, exercise, and seeing a psychologist or other professional. A study recently completed found that the Mediterranean diet improved the mood of people suffering depression[131]. Medication should really be just a temporary solution, and what you need is a long-term solution.

MAY'S STORY

May's father died the day before her daughter was born. May was twenty-four years old. Initially, no one told her about his death.

She was in hospital and he was in the mortuary. Eventually she found out. She went into a deep depression, as she had been very close to her father. People ignored her and didn't know what to do. Her doctor referred her to a psychiatrist. She went for a consultation with the psychiatrist, but walked out, as it didn't feel right. She was suffering from a combination of post-natal depression and depression related to grief. It took her seven years to get over it by herself.

The take-away from this story is that attempting to fix yourself can take a great deal longer than getting help from a professional who is a good fit for you.

The reasons for depression can be complex, and so taking control of your own treatment and approach, and finding the best counsellor, psychologist or particular treatment for you is a very important aspect of recovery.

GRIEF AND LOSS

As we go through life there are times when we will experience grief. Events may occur that have a negative impact on us. Whether you are unemployed and can't find work, you lose your job, have a relationship break up, lose a friendship, or experience the death of a loved one, it is very normal to feel depressed and sad for a while.

Grief is a natural process and is not a mental illness. It is quite ok to feel sad, down, and unhappy, but it is important to go through the grieving process and work through your emotions and thoughts about your loss so that you can eventually feel more balanced about life.

When a loss is experienced, the intensity of the grief reflects the relationship, so that generally speaking, the closer the relationship with the person or thing, the greater the impact of the loss.

Everyone grieves in their own way, and there are large differences from person to person. You might find that you are expressive and that you cry a lot, or you just might feel a profound sadness. Both of these responses, and all the possible behaviours in between, are fine. At the beginning, you will be in shock and probably feel numb, and you may initially disbelieve the news.

Numbness may last a short time or longer, but eventually the reality of the situation is accepted—at least on a mental level. After the shock of the loss has worn off, a large range of emotions and thoughts may arise for you. Anger, sadness, grief, and loneliness are common. During the next six weeks or longer emotions come up and symptoms may occur, such as difficulty sleeping, loss of concentration, thoughts of the person you have lost, and many others. The reality of the loss also needs to be accepted on an emotional level during this time[132].

Psychologist J. William Worden suggests that there are four tasks that people need to traverse when experiencing a loss.

The first task is to accept the reality of the loss. This occurs on two levels, mentally and emotionally.

The second task is to process the pain of loss.

The third is to adjust to a world in which the deceased is missing.

The fourth is to find a continuing bond with the deceased while embarking on a new life[133].

While these tasks are specifically for people experiencing the loss of a loved one, the tasks are actually equally true for any other type of loss. For instance, if you lost your job then you would need to accept the reality of that loss, to experience the pain of that loss, to adjust to a world in which you no longer have that job, and then to move on, despite the fact that you lost your job, so that you may find another job or otherwise embark on a new life and find new beginnings.

The most important point about grief is that it is an entirely normal reaction. Everyone grieves in their own unique way. You may find that you can manage to go through your mourning process by yourself, with just the help of a supportive social network. Otherwise, you may find that asking for help in some way will allow you to manage the process more easily.

There are online resources, there are grief support groups available either online or in person, and there is individual counselling with a psychologist or counsellor, which you may find of benefit. Things that may make your grief more difficult or complicated to process include the suddenness of the loss, the closeness of the relationship, a number of losses in a reasonably short time span, trauma aspects and unexpectedness. When you experience many losses in a short time frame including different losses, this can also complicate matters and mean that processing everything can be difficult by yourself.

Reaching out for help is a good strategy. Visit www.dianahutchison.com for some ideas. See the third book in this series, *A Practical Guide for Grief and Loss.*

ANXIETY

Everyone experiences anxiety, but some people experience it more than others and then the anxiety can become debilitating.

We all have anxiety over how we'll go in tests at school, or when we need to perform well, such as in job interviews.

Some people experience anxiety in social situations, while others have a fear of public speaking. Every individual is different. If we are anxious, we worry about an issue or event. Often our worries don't eventuate. However, that doesn't mean that it is necessarily easy to stop worrying.

In our current world of connectedness and technology, there are new fears and anxieties emerging. One in particular is the "Fear of Missing Out" (FOMO).

This is the fear of exclusion from what's happening, often in relation to your friends and peers. This fear contributes to people checking their phones constantly, and a difficulty with being disconnected for any length of time.

An Australian Psychological Society survey carried out in 2015[134] found that one in ten Australians reported that keeping up with social media networks was a source of stress for them. It also found that social media can reduce stress, with about 57% of Australians reporting this effect.

Social media dominates the lives of Australian teens. More than half of all teens find it difficult to relax or sleep after spending time on social media, and 60% feel brain burnout from constant connectivity. Half of all teens experience FOMO[135], while a quarter of adults' experience FOMO. You would be at risk for FOMO if you believe the following:

- It is important that friends' in-jokes are understood.

- Your friends are having more rewarding experiences than you.

- It isn't ok for your friends to have fun without you.

- Missing out on planned get-togethers is something to worry about.

If you spend a lot of time on social media and would like to reduce that amount of time, then this is likely to be of benefit. Be aware that your life is not just on your phone. While there are benefits using your phone in relation to finding information and connecting with people, it can certainly be a time-waster too. Consider what other things you can be doing instead of endless scrolling, with the possibility of becoming even more anxious.

It could be more beneficial for your mental health to be connecting with more people face-to-face, or going with your friends to places where you can be in natural surroundings, such as a park, the beach, or reserve. Even places like the Botanical Gardens provide nature and also the options for refreshments and discussions. Trees and gardens give you the mental and spiritual uplift you may require to release anxiety and stress. Research shows that being in nature is beneficial for health and wellbeing[136].

When you are studying or working, see whether it is possible to check your phone during breaks—the rest of the time, pay attention and focus on the activity you are engaged in. A challenge for you could be to keep on reducing the number of times you check your phone until you get to a point where you are checking no more than once per hour. You could start by making the gaps between checking progressively longer, moving from ten minutes to twenty minutes and so on, up to one hour. This may be somewhat difficult, but persist! You may find that distracting yourself works best.

There are positive benefits to social media, as well as negative aspects. Social media is a good tool to connect you with your loved ones at a distance, to join groups you are interested in, to find out information, and to share interests with a community. This especially true when meeting in-person with those people or those you care about is just not feasible.

With online platforms in the business space becoming more widely used, and with online meetings easier to organise and hold, the ways we connect with others, both personally and professionally, have changed forever.

PANIC ATTACKS

If you have a panic attack, you may experience the following symptoms:

- You feel that you could be having a heart attack.

- You think you are going to die.

- You have uncontrollable urges to go to the toilet.

- You need to get out of the situation you are in as fast as possible.

The best way to manage a panic attack is to breathe slowly or even to hold your breath for a little while. If your breathing speeds up, as commonly happens when you are anxious, then you hyperventilate and feel even worse. So, breathe slowly, tell yourself you are not going to die, you are not having a heart attack, you are going to be fine, and that you can get through this time. Breathe in for the count of 5, hold for 5, breathe out for the count of 5 and hold for 5. This will reduce the feeling of dizziness which comes with hyperventilating and excess oxygen. It also calms your physical response of your body overall. It is likely that your main thought at this time is to get out of the situation where you are and get to a place of safety.

The most effective way of treating panic attacks is to find a professional or a program that incorporates cognitive behavioural therapy (CBT) and/or exposure therapy at the same time. This means that you navigate increasingly difficult situations as you put yourself in increasingly more stressful situations. After you have successfully navigated the first situation, you go to the next one. Your treatment may also include some cognitive behavioural therapy, to help you challenge the beliefs and thoughts that you have when in a situation that causes the panic response. Other kinds of treatments may also be beneficial such as hypnosis, and NLP.

GENERALISED ANXIETY DISORDER

Generalised anxiety disorder is a condition where the person feels anxious about a number of different things. There is no focus for the anxiety, except the future and what it might hold for oneself and for others. Generalised anxiety disorder can be very difficult.

To live perpetually in dread and fear is very harmful to the body since the "fight or flight" response is continually triggered, and so the body becomes stressed. This can then cause further illness through the immune system being compromised. Generalised anxiety disorder also creates an intolerance for uncertainty and a need for reassurance from others.

One point to note is that life is *inherently uncertain*. The more you can bring yourself to the present moment—the now—the less you will be projecting yourself into the future (or the past).

A number of treatments may be useful for someone with generalised anxiety disorder. Cognitive behavioural therapy delivered by a psychologist may be beneficial. Other processes that may work are mindfulness, meditation, and hypnosis. If you have anxiety, you need to relearn how to think about events in life, and to find more adaptive strategies to approaching the future. If you have generalised anxiety disorder, then finding the right treatment for you will help you become less anxious.

In addition, have an exploration of your diet. The Mediterranean diet has been shown to help anxiety as well as depression. You could also check out whether you have any food sensitivities or intolerances, as some research has shown that probiotics can be beneficial.

EATING DISORDERS

Two common eating disorders are anorexia nervosa and bulimia nervosa[137].

In anorexia, the sufferer puts strict controls on how much food and sometimes how much water they take in. There is a particularly high risk of fatality with this disorder[138].

In bulimia, there is a pattern of gorging and purging, so that the sufferer loses the nutrition that would otherwise be provided by the food eaten.

Both of these conditions may affect both sexes at any age. However, they appear to be most common among young people.

Anxiety about body image often affects girls and boys, where social media and advertising communicate what society sees as the "ideal body". Concern about eating can start off slowly but end up as anorexia or bulimia.

With anorexia nervosa, the individual may take in such a small amount of food that long-term health effects occur. Provided the sufferer gets appropriate treatment, these negative effects may be reduced. The sufferer may not just starve him or herself, but may engage in huge amounts of exercise as well. This is all in the name of becoming the "ideal" weight. One aspect of the disorder is that sufferers have a very distorted view of themselves and what they look like.

With bulimia, there is a pattern of binge eating followed by purging—whether by forcing oneself to vomit or through the use of laxatives. This means that very little of the food is absorbed by the body. The vomiting may be seen as a self-punishment for eating. For a recovery story from bulimia see the book, *My Name is Caroline*[139].

Societal norms of the "ideal body", combined with images used in advertising, marketing and social media, have some input into sufferers' experiences. This means the more discussion there is in the home around the ideas about how unrealistic the "ideal body" is, the better. Young people who have not yet reached puberty do not yet have their adult body shape. In fact, body shape is fluid until the late teens and early twenties. Discussion around such concepts may be helpful. If you feel anxiety about your body image, then continue reading and see particularly the section on body image in the chapter on self-esteem.

Treatment of eating disorders requires ongoing support and belief-changing therapy through an eating disorders program. Another option would be cognitive behavioural therapy with an experienced psychologist. Alternatively, you could try NLP. In this way, you can target the beliefs directly and change them. The important thing is to have such treatment under the supervision of a medical doctor.

AVOIDANT RESTRICTIVE FOOD INTAKE DISORDER (ARFID)

ARFID is another eating disorder[140]. It is similar to anorexia in relation to the limitations in the amount or type of food consumed, but unlike anorexia it doesn't involve any distress about body size or fears of being fat. There may, however, be fear of choking or fear of eating new foods. ARFID is characterised by highly selective eating habits, which may be based on the colours or textures of food.

While children may go through phases of picky eating, a person with ARFID doesn't consume enough food to grow and develop normally, so that stalled weight and growth may occur. In adults, not enough food is consumed to maintain basic body function. Supplements could be the only way to enable nutrition to be maintained.

Problems may arise at school and work due to psychosocial issues, including concerns about eating with others[141]. The best thing to do is to get treatment from a trained professional. Treatment does help to alleviate the issues.

BINGE EATING DISORDER

Binge eating disorder is similar to bulimia, without the purging behaviour. Often, food is binged on even when the person isn't hungry.

Food may be eaten to forget thoughts and feelings. However, feelings of depression, guilt and disgust may arise after the binging behaviour. The person may engage in sporadic fasts and repetitive diets in response to the negative feelings evoked. Binging is often done secretly and alone.

Approximately 47% of people with an eating disorder suffer from binge eating disorder[142]. Low self-esteem is common, as is a negative body image.

If you think this is what you have then seeking treatment is your best option. A psychologist, counsellor or NLP practitioner may be helpful.

ORTHOREXIA NERVOSA

This is a disorder that may develop from healthy eating patterns [143]. If you are a healthy diet enthusiast and develop anxiety around eating healthily then this may turn into a problem.

A problem might be beginning if you have the following:

• That your healthy eating is taking up a lot of your time and is interfering with your daily life.

• Eating any food you regard as unhealthy leaves you feeling anxious and impure.

• Your sense of peace and sense of self is based on the purity and rightness of the food you eat.

• You have gradually decreased the number of foods that you feel are healthy for you.

• Your health has deteriorated since you have begun to place more focus on your diet[144].

If you have become obsessed with healthy eating and will go to great lengths to ensure you are eating healthily and can say yes to any of the above, then think about taking some action to reduce your obsession. While it is good to have a balanced diet and to eat healthy food, there is a point at which it becomes too much. It is important to remain balanced, rather than go to the extremes.

In this case, a "good-enough" healthy diet is ideal. Where you allow yourself the occasional unhealthy food and cannot identify an obsession with healthy eating then you are likely to be just fine. Otherwise, find a professional who can help you.

PHOBIAS

People can also develop phobias through intense anxiety.

A phobia is an irrational fear of a specific object, whether this is an animal or a thing. Usually, there is an event when the thing or object first produced anxiety and fear. Subsequently, there is an irrational fear that is evoked whenever the object is perceived.

Such examples may be spiders, snakes, lizards, dogs, fear of heights, fear of public speaking, and so on. These are simple phobias, which usually develop in childhood. In treatment, a good approach is cognitive behavioural therapy using graduated exposure treatment. Alternatively, another treatment for simple phobias is NLP.

There are also a wide number of more complex phobias, including social phobia and agoraphobia (fear of open spaces).

SOCIAL PHOBIA

People can develop social phobia where they get anxious in social situations. While many of us may get anxious in social situations when we meet new people, it becomes debilitating when your anxiety goes way up and you find you need to get out of the situation.

Meeting new people is not the only situation that those suffering social anxiety find difficult. There are also situations such as using public transport or going shopping in supermarkets or malls.

Meeting peoples' eyes can be problematic as well. This means that it can limit one's lifestyle and reduce social outings and connection. St Vincent's hospital in Sydney has a good program for social phobia, and the program is also available online[145].

Treatment involves putting yourself in situations that become gradually more difficult, and becoming acclimatised to them. In this way, you become comfortable with each level as you go up in the order of difficulty. In reality, it is exposure therapy. Hypnosis with imagery rehearsal could also be helpful.

AGORAPHOBIA

Agoraphobia is a fear of open spaces, and often those who have it can't go very far from their home. Being housebound can be particularly debilitating to one's life and what one can achieve. Again, NLP can be helpful, as can a combination of cognitive behavioural therapy and hypnosis, as well as exposure therapy. Finding a good psychologist or therapist who will visit your home is crucial, as is addressing all the psychological aspects related to the condition.

If someone you know experiences anxiety or a phobia of some kind, it isn't helpful to tell them to just get over it. The anxiety is an automatic response that is hard-wired in the brain. There are ways of loosening the connections, but it often takes time and specific techniques.

POST-TRAUMATIC STRESS DISORDER

Post-Traumatic Stress Disorder (PTSD) may come about when a person suffers an extraordinary loss, witnesses or experiences one or more traumatic events, has been in a life-threatening situation, or experiences a man-made or natural disaster.

Multiple events that are deemed by the person to be traumatic and upsetting may also lead to PTSD. Additionally, people may also be traumatised through hearing about many experiences of trauma. There is now more recognition of how trauma may be experienced and realistically includes a wider range of situations and is becoming more of a self-diagnosis. This means that depending on the person's experience of trauma, the diagnosis may be appropriate in a wider range of situations than outlined in previous times.

Symptoms may include re-experiencing the traumatic event in dreams or flashbacks, hypervigilance, avoidance of anything connected with the trauma, being easily startled, and numbness. It sometimes helps to talk about the trauma, and prolonged exposure also helps (imagining it in their mind). See The Black Dog Institute website for information and options for treatment[146].

Psychological counselling with a specialist in trauma may be appropriate. There is also an online course available through St Vincent's Hospital, Sydney[147].

Alternatively, cognitive behavioural therapy is appropriate and, in addition, there is Eye Movement and Desensitisation Reprocessing (EMDR), which can be administered by a psychologist who has had the correct training. Both CBT and EMDR treatments are evidence-based. There are other modalities that may also be effective. It is a matter of seeing what works best for you.

Research has continued in this area, and practices such as yoga and mindfulness have been shown to be effective in helping trauma sufferers. Pet therapy and equine therapy can also be helpful, and it is likely that engaging in creative expression within a therapeutic environment is effective too[148]. Art therapy is beneficial for a number of conditions, not just PTSD. Other treatments may also be available.

OBSESSIVE COMPULSIVE DISORDER

In obsessive compulsive disorder (OCD), the obsession is the thought or image that recurs, and the compulsion is the ritual or act that is performed to neutralise the thought.

Checking and cleaning are common[149]. Often, the checking or cleaning needs to be absolutely perfect before the thought is negated, so a lot of time can be taken up in these rituals, and the impact on daily living can be enormous. Treatment may involve exposure and response prevention, which is behaviour therapy, or some people may respond to cognitive behavioural therapy. There are some specific treatment centres available, so explore in your area for these services.

PSYCHOSES

Psychotic illnesses (such as bipolar disorder or schizophrenia) often start in the late teens and early twenties when stress may be experienced in one's life, although they can be detected earlier at times[150].

Psychotic illnesses can also start later in life. If your family has some members who have had a psychotic illness then you have a greater risk of being affected yourself. Even so, it is not a huge risk, and don't forget that environmental circumstances need to kick off the gene expression that you may or may not have.

This means that factors such as stress, age, and what is ingested or inhaled, can spark off an episode of psychosis. A number of drugs can also cause psychosis[151].

Evidence is coming to light about the connection between the gut and the brain, and the many different ways that the microbiome may be impacting inflammation in the body, which can lead to chronic inflammation that can go to the brain[152]. What this means is that, over time, diet and microbiota in the gut could be causing the psychosis through a build-up of inflammation in the brain. This is therefore an avenue of exploration, particularly when psychosis occurs later in life, where there are no other reasons found.

BIPOLAR DISORDER

Bipolar is a mood disorder in which a person cycles between mania (feeling euphoric) and depression (feeling very down).

In mania, the thoughts are fast, and fantasy may play a large role so that the person can get themselves in all sorts of trouble. The depression can be so low that the person can become dangerously suicidal.

The cycling through these two states can be reasonably fast in terms of weeks, or slow, with a number of months in each state. One of the drugs used to treat bipolar disorder is lithium, which, if first taken when in a manic state, helps the person to balance out. Some people stop taking their medication because they don't like not feeling the way they feel when in the manic state. As a result, medication compliance can be an issue for people with bipolar disorder. Medication may relieve most of the symptoms of psychosis, but it is not a cure.

Taking medication for the rest of your life could be one option to consider. This could be an immediate and best option while you are investigating other possibilities for improving your wellbeing, such as diet, reducing stress, and exploring mindfulness. It is important to consider there *may* be a genetic factor playing a role. However, exploring self-healing possibilities for improving your quality of life will be beneficial. This could include working on your mindset and stress levels, addressing any physical issues, in order to become healthier overall. This can, at the very least, reduce the effects of the condition on your life.

It is always a good idea to find out the possible side effects of the drug being suggested: the fewer side effects, the better. However, everyone has their own unique body chemistry, so different drugs may affect different people in specific ways. This is why it may take some time to find the drug that works the best for you.

SCHIZOPHRENIA

The other major psychotic illness is schizophrenia. This is a thought disorder and when in the throes of an episode there is often delusional thinking and visual hallucinations.

Usually, there are voices in one's head that are experienced as real and outside of the self. What will be experienced is very specific to the individual.

There is a distinction between schizophrenia and paranoid schizophrenia. In the paranoid version there are often delusions of persecution. If there are no persecution beliefs, then a diagnosis of schizophrenia may be given. In this event, there may be delusional beliefs of being a world saviour or something similar. There may be religious overtones or there may not. In any case, the delusions tend to be consistent with the worldview and personality of the sufferer, so they are unique. Since the delusions and hallucinations are experienced as reality, the person's behaviour may be bizarre to the outsider. If, for instance, you believe that animals are saying nasty things to you, then you may try to avoid them. If you believe that there are cameras everywhere and that you are on the Internet (when this is not the case in reality) then it is likely that you will behave in a way that is congruent with this belief. It can be extremely frightening for the person suffering with the delusions, and for those around them.

Contrary to popular belief, schizophrenia is not a split personality. Rather, it is a thought disorder that adheres strongly to the conscious and unconscious mind of the sufferer.

Since bizarre behaviour gets noticed by families, and sometimes by the authorities, such behaviour may lead to treatment. Some drugs have been developed which are beneficial in symptom relief. Again, it might be necessary to try different medications until you find the right one, or the right combination. If your psychiatrist does not have an empathic view and does not allow you to try the more recent drugs, and if you are having bad side effects, please get a second opinion from a different psychiatrist.

Should you come off the medication some time after the first episode and have another psychotic episode, then this could indicate that a longer time on medication may be necessary.

It is beneficial to have psychological counselling even if you have a psychiatrist who is supervising your medication. Some psychiatrists are very traditional and do not enter into any psychotherapy kind of treatment. Others, however, do. If you are lucky enough to have a psychiatrist who is more progressive, and can provide multi-level treatments, this is likely to help a great deal. However, if you make progress in relation to your mental health, through working with a psychologist and focus not only on your mental health, but also on other life aspects, including diet, stress levels and lifestyle factors, you are likely to have a much better outcome in the long term. It is important not to suddenly stop medication. This is because sudden withdrawal of your medication can spark off symptoms[153]. For this reason, it is important to gradually reduce the dosage where possible and be monitored properly. This may take a year or more to do, but in this case, there is a greatly reduced risk of a relapse occurring.

It is a good idea to be under a good psychiatrist for a reasonable time, because they are experienced in treating mental illness and psychoses. A normal medical doctor or General Practitioner (GP) is not qualified to treat these things, so ensure you get a referral to a psychiatrist. GPs may be reliable in prescribing antidepressants for depression, but it would be safer to get a referral to see a psychiatrist in the first instance.

There is some evidence that regular marijuana use may trigger schizophrenia in some people[154]. The inhalation of this drug would therefore be seen as an environmental factor that triggers the condition in those who are susceptible. Therefore, should schizophrenia be in your family history, then it could be an idea to stay away from marijuana.

STIGMA

Mental illness may be temporary or it may last a longer time. There is more public recognition and acceptance of it now than there used to be. Well-known people have begun to be more open about their experiences with mental illness and mental health struggles, so there is less stigma associated with it now—although there is still some way to go before there is full acceptance within society.

MANAGING A MENTAL ILLNESS

It is important to find the best ways to manage your mental illness. It is healthier not to let your mental illness define who you are. You are a person who has values, needs, and desires, who just *happens* to also have a mental illness.

You are not your mental illness.

You are more than your mental illness. While talking about your troubles, breakdowns, and so on may be beneficial sometimes, if you talk about these things at every opportunity then you are letting your illness define who you are. You are more than your latest episode. Instead of always talking about your illness, talk about things such as your goals and hobbies, what you'd like to do, and your dreams.

Wherever you are at, it is important to keep yourself safe. Recognise the triggers for your issue and find a professional who can help you manage your mental health. Ensure you ask medical professionals about the side effects of any medicine. The fewer the side effects suffered, the better. There are now some effective medications available.

Where you have been told that you need to be on the medication for the rest of your life, it is wise to heed this advice. Just because you feel better when on the medication doesn't indicate that the problem is fixed. It is just that the symptoms are under control with the medication. As previously mentioned, if you have done the work on yourself—physically, mentally, and emotionally, and have changed your diet and lifestyle, then you can always check with a good health professional and slowly reduce medication where appropriate.

No matter what the mental health issue is, it is important to find support. A psychiatrist could be the first support, and it would be important to also find a psychologist or counsellor to talk with. They could help you manage your emotions, and discussion around thoughts and feelings may be very beneficial for you. In addition, they will be able to help you decide on the best coping strategies that will stand you in good stead through this time. Discussion about your life, lifestyle, mindset, beliefs and values could be helpful—including finding and exploring your goals, purpose, and how to achieve these. Taking action in these areas may turn your life around.

It is helpful to find activities that you enjoy and engage in them. This will be a beneficial approach to management. One thing likely to be of benefit is being in nature. Whether this entails going for walks or simply being in a garden or green space, surrounding yourself with plants and living things can be very healing. There has been greater recognition of the healing aspect of gardens in recent times for both physical and mental issues. Being in nature is grounding and lifts the spirits. Getting out into nature, particularly where there are plants or water, will be soothing and relaxing.

RECOVERING FROM A MENTAL ILLNESS

The best reason for being on medication is to alleviate symptoms while you are engaging in treatment that has been shown to be helpful in the long term. This can include behaviour therapy for phobias and anxiety, cognitive behaviour therapy for depression and OCD, and specific programs for eating disorders and OCD. Once treatment has been completed, then the medication may be reduced and stopped under the supervision of your doctor.

If you have had a mental health issue for a long time, then recovering may present some difficulties. Since you will be used to behaving in certain ways and thinking certain thoughts, there is likely to be a time of transition to being free to behave in different ways. It may feel strange or unsettling. Using a gratitude journal, engaging in activities you enjoy, relaxing, resting, living more in the present, and being able to forgive yourself and others may all be helpful in this process[155].

Replace the nervousness that you may feel, and label it as excitement. Then you may manage this time better. Be excited about what you might discover about where you are now. Notice what is different and be happy with the positive changes. Go with the flow. This is the new you. Take a few low-level risks, such as socialising with friends in a safe situation without drugs or alcohol, and see how that feels. Behave as you would like to behave, taking into account how you were before this issue came up for you. If there's anything you want to change, now is the ideal time to start putting those changes into place.

With mental health issues, the thing that gets knocked around most is your self-esteem. Take time to be kind to yourself, surround yourself with people who lift you up. Build up your self-esteem. Work on building a skill, getting better at some activity, and building relationships. You can do these things whether or not you have recovered from your illness. This is also part of the management process. Engaging in counselling should also be beneficial.

> **STRATEGIES TO IMPROVE MENTAL HEALTH, WELLBEING, AND RESILIENCE**
>
> Gratitude
>
> Empathy
>
> Mindfulness
>
> Being in the present moment
>
> Self-love
>
> See the book *The Resilience Project*[156]
>
> Ask yourself, 'What went well today?'
>
> Through using these strategies, you will create improvements in your ability to cope when things aren't going well.

RECOGNISING MENTAL ILLNESS

How do you recognise mental illness in yourself or in someone else?

This list is not exhaustive, but there are a few things to watch out for:

- Withdrawing from social interaction, isolating yourself

- Thoughts of self-harm, feeling hopeless, helpless and depressed
- Engaging in unusual behaviours
- Having moments of staring off into space
- Concern about persecution
- Preoccupation with food
- Concern about being fat, when not
- Fears/behaviours interfering with living
- Talking fast, doing everything fast, getting into trouble, spending money
- Getting into trouble with the police, when not usually criminal
- Talking about God, the devil, demons or angels in unusual contexts

SUMMARY

- Be aware that everyone experiences times in their lives where they feel down, depressed or anxious.

- Consider finding some treatment if your thoughts and emotions change from how you used to be (in a negative direction).

- Seek counselling if you are having difficulties with experiencing the loss of someone or something, in order to help you through the grieving and mourning process.

- Get treatment for anxiety, especially if it is adversely affecting your life.

- Don't be afraid to ask for help.

- Take time to find the right person to help you and seek second opinions.

- Wean yourself off social media, or get help, if you feel you have FOMO.

- Consider NLP as a treatment for phobias.

- Acknowledge that you are more than your illness, and that you are more than your thoughts and behaviour. You are still a unique human being and should accept that you are still awesome. If you suspect you are bipolar or schizophrenic or if you are diagnosed with these conditions, then get treatment.

- Find the right program or the right psychologist to treat eating disorders. Don't delay. It's important to get treatment due to the rate of fatalities, especially with anorexia nervosa. By getting the right treatment you will find that you end up with a much better quality of life than you would otherwise have.

- Always consider self-help options to improve your life in conjunction with any kind of therapy, such as dancing, singing, support groups, yoga, mindfulness, meditation, and exercise.

- Remember you are not alone.

- By taking these steps can become awesome at managing your mental health.

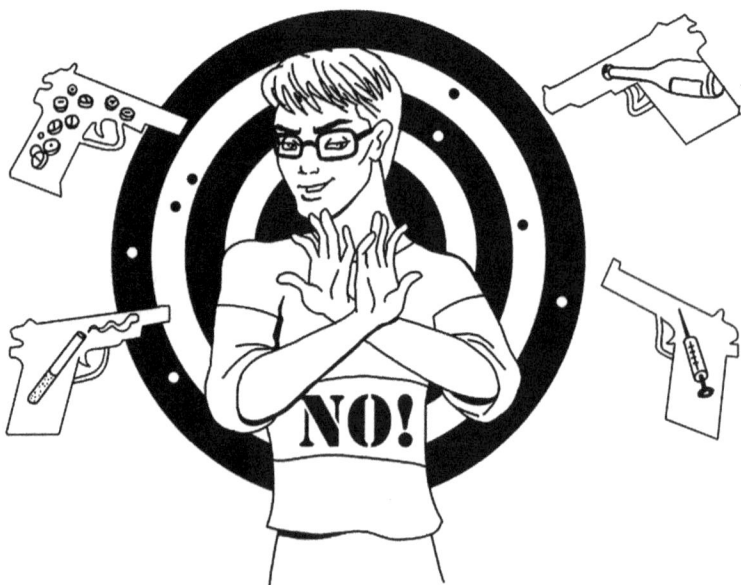

CHAPTER 11

ADDICTIONS

What is at the root of your addiction?

Addictions may involve physical dependence on a substance, and/or a psychological dependence.

In the brain, the reward system is triggered when we behave in a certain way, for instance ingesting a particular substance, and we can become addicted to chasing this initial feeling. Some substances are very addictive, while others are less so.

Sometimes one person may become addicted, while another may not. It is a very individual response, since we all have unique brain chemistry and unique ways of thinking about things that may influence our behaviour when it comes to addictions.

If you find you are addicted to something that is causing you problems in some way, you can take steps to rehabilitate yourself and change. Whether you manage this by yourself or with help will depend on your specific addiction and your past history in relation to it. You may wish to consider the underlying reasons why you might be addicted. *What are you self-medicating for?*

Sometimes, treating the underlying issues or reasons means that you can stop the addiction more easily. If you are young, are having a difficult time at present, and are in crisis in some way, then check out the Martin Foundation[157]. On occasions, swapping for a better and more positive substitute can also help in the process of recovery.

COMMON ADDICTIONS

The substances that people most commonly become addicted to and dependent on that cause major problems are alcohol, nicotine, and drugs.

Each substance can be difficult to withdraw from, and it takes a great amount of determination and effort. However, it is possible, and all is not lost if you are addicted. There is hope. As with any addiction or dependence, the more you work on stopping, the more likely you are to succeed. It's about finding the strategies that are effective for you.

There has been some discussion over the years as to whether there is such a thing as an addictive personality. The thinking is that someone with an addictive personality has a higher likelihood of developing an addiction. There may be something in this, but it is by no means set in stone. The debate is not especially helpful however you look at it. What we do know is that factors such as availability and peer pressure are key components for people to experiment with—and even to continue taking—a particular substance[158]. There are many other factors too, including internal characteristics, and social and cultural aspects.

With most addictive substances, and particularly drugs, there is a "high" when you initially take the substance. People may become addicted from the first rush. However, the body quickly becomes used to the substance, and so a greater quantity is required to feel the high, and even to feel normal. As a result, there is a continual searching to recapture the feeling that came from the first high.

With substance use and abuse, there is often what is called a "secondary gain". This means that you get something out of taking the substance that essentially keeps you on the path of taking it. So, for instance, with alcohol, the effect can help you feel more relaxed and less inhibited. If you are a bit anxious in social settings, then the relaxing effect of alcohol will help to maintain the desire to drink when you are socialising. In addition, with alcohol and other socially accepted drugs, there is also the peer pressure element that continues to maintain this behaviour. However, addiction takes this further and is more destructive to you, your relationships, and the wider community.

ALCOHOL

There is No Safe Amount of Any Drug, Including Alcohol.

In 2020-2021, one in four Australians over 18 years of age, drank more than the recommended amount, either on a daily or weekly basis. Alcohol is the most widely used drug[159]. (These figures are Australia-wide and are from Australian Bureau of Statistics figures)

In 2022, the alcohol-induced death rate was the highest it's been in 10 years[160].

Australians have the highest intake per capita of alcohol in relation to the OECD countries.

Alcohol can have toxic effects on your body. It is classified as a group 1 carcinogen by the IARC, which means it causes cancer. Cancers particularly related to alcohol are those of the mouth, throat, tongue, and liver.

Excessive alcohol consumption is a cause of a wide range of health issues and other harms, including being the major cause of road accidents, domestic and public violence, crime, liver disease, and brain damage, as well as contributing to family breakdown and broader social dysfunction.

'Lifetime risky drinkers' are those who consume more than *two* standard drinks per day. 'Single occasion risky drinkers' are those who consume *four or more* standard drinks on one occasion.

The more you drink, and the more often you drink, the higher your risk for alcohol-related diseases and death.

Alcohol is a nervous system depressant. It has been associated with a range of diseases that may cause death and adverse effects that reduce the quality of life. These include: cardiovascular disease, cancers, diabetes, nutrition related disorders, excess weight and obesity, risks to unborn babies, liver diseases, mental health conditions such as depression and anxiety, dependency, long term cognitive impairment, and self-harm.

If you have a large amount of alcohol, you could overdose.

Call an ambulance straight away by dialling triple zero (000) if you or someone else has any of the following symptoms (ambulance officers don't need to involve the police):

- confusion
- blurred vision
- clumsiness
- memory loss
- nausea or vomiting
- passing out
- coma
- death

Long-term effects

Regular use of alcohol may eventually cause:

- depression
- poor memory and brain damage
- difficulty getting an erection

- difficulty having children
- liver disease
- cancer
- high blood pressure and heart disease
- needing to drink more to get the same effect
- physical dependence on alcohol

see https://www.adf.org.au[161]

Twelve conditions linked
to chronic heavy drinking

- Anaemia
- Cancer
- Cardiovascular disease
- Cirrhosis of the liver
- Dementia
- Depression
- Seizures
- Gout
- High blood pressure
- Infectious diseases, due to immune system being suppressed
- Nerve damage
- Pancreatitis
- Death

For more information see https://www.drinkfacts.com.au

There is growing evidence that alcohol has serious adverse effects on growing brains. Since the brain is still growing up to the age of twenty-five then, ideally, you should limit your alcohol use until after this age. Of course, even after this age, copious amounts of alcohol are still going to damage your brain and your health[162].

Both binge drinking and daily drinking are problematic. However, because drinking in Australia continues to be a large part of the culture, there may be an issue for you in the situation where you stop drinking but still socialise with your friends. There is more recognition now about the effects of alcohol, and people may be more tolerant of others not drinking. If you decide to go down this path then while it may test some of your friendships, it may be very good for your health.

In the situation where you decide to limit your drinking, but not to stop completely, then you can limit your intake to no more than four standard drinks on one occasion. And if you are drinking daily, then limit your consumption to one to two standard drinks with a break of two to four days per week.

When it comes to drinking and driving, society is now more accepting of not drinking when driving, and will applaud self-responsibility in this situation. It's much better to be completely sober when driving. Work out who will be the designated driver when you are planning to go out with friends.

In order to resist the peer pressure that you may experience, it is important to have made up your mind beforehand as to where your limit is. So, whether you are not drinking alcohol at all or only having one drink, have this limit in your head. It will probably be easier if you substitute a non-alcoholic drink for an alcoholic one, rather than not drinking anything at all. When others are buying rounds, ask for an orange juice, for example. If you have some good reasons for not drinking, then you can wheel them out when people ask you. To some degree, in order to reduce the peer pressure, you just need to keep seeing it as an individual choice.

When it comes down to it, there is only going to be a certain amount of pressure put on you, and so you just need to be able to say no for longer than the pressure is exerted. See it as the best action you can take for you. You are not stopping others from enjoying themselves. And you aren't stopping yourself from having a good time, either. You'll just be in a much better space in the morning and over the long term.

If you make a decision before you go out that you will only have two drinks, and then drink non-alcoholic drinks after that, then you will be able to enjoy yourself much more.

You'll be able to remember everything, you'll be able to make better decisions, and you'll be less likely to end up in trouble, as well as have better short and long-term health outcomes.

MEGAN'S STORY

One night after work, Megan went to the local pub and drank four cocktails. After that, she was the drunkest she'd ever been. Everything was blurred, she couldn't walk straight, and she couldn't talk straight. She left the pub by herself, and had to cross the main road to get home. The next day, she had no recollection of how she crossed the road, but she had managed to find her way home. When she got home, she went to bed. The room was spinning round and round and she felt extremely sick. The following morning, she had a blinding hangover. From this experience, Megan decided that she would only have a couple of drinks at any one sitting. Since that time, she has kept to her decision pretty well, only having up to three glasses of wine at any one time. She has never been so drunk again.

TOBACCO

Nicotine is a very addictive drug. Smoking has many negative effects, and very few positives.

Cigarette smoke contains over seventy carcinogens that may cause cancer[163], as well as damage to the heart and circulatory system.

Lung cancer is a big possibility, as well as heart disease, and a number of respiratory diseases including emphysema. It not only affects the health of the smoker, but also of those around them. In this time of plain packaging in Australia there is possibly less peer pressure now to smoke than in the past. And there are fewer places where one can smoke in the public arena.

Regular smoking of tobacco products which contain nicotine has well-documented negative effects on health and is recognised as a major preventable cause of premature death and disability around the world[164]. Use of nicotine through smoking may eventually cause the following types of chronic disease and issues:
- stroke
- blindness, cataracts (eye diseases)
- birth defects if the foetus is exposed to cigarettes
- periodontitis (yellowing teeth, gum disease)

- aortic aneurism (enlarging of major blood vessels)
- coronary heart disease
- pneumonia
- various respiratory diseases (shortness of breath, asthma, coughing fits)
- diabetes
- reduced fertility
- ectopic pregnancy
- hip fractures
- male sexual dysfunction
- rheumatoid arthritis
- reduced immune function (regular colds and flu)
- overall diminished health (ageing, back pain, slower-healing wounds, mood swings)
- dependence on smoking
- financial, work, and social problems.

See: https://www.adf.org.au/drugfacts/nicotine

If you do smoke, then the sooner and faster you manage to quit, the better your health outcomes will be. The added bonus is the extra money you will have, which you can either save or spend on things that are not damaging to your health. The more times you try to quit, the more likely it is that you will be able to stop for good. It is important to work out what issues you will have when quitting, and the best ways to deal with them.

- Twelve hours after stopping, almost all nicotine is out of your system, with most by-products gone within five days.

- After twenty-four hours, the level of carbon monoxide in your blood has dropped dramatically, meaning your body can take and use oxygen more efficiently.

- After two days, your senses of taste and smell start to return.

- After two months, blood flow to your hands and feet improves.

- After one year, your risk of heart disease rapidly drops.

- After ten years, your risk of lung cancer is halved.[165]

When I was quitting smoking, I found that I needed to give myself permission to eat biscuits instead of doing the hand to mouth action that I had done when smoking. That was a fairly big thing for me. So, there I was watching television, scoffing biscuits by the packet. I put on about seven kilos, but after a few months I stopped eating biscuits and went back to my original weight.

I also found that reading was good, because it took my mind off any cravings and took me to another reality. You can work out the best strategies to get through the cravings and try different ones each time you try to quit, so that the best one may come about on the ultimate attempt.

Once you get past the first three days, then you can look forward to three weeks, then three months, then one year and then longer. You can reward yourself for doing a good job by saving up the money that you would have otherwise spent on cigarettes and spending it on something that is healthier, such as going to the movies, going out to dinner, or some other treat that you would enjoy.

One point to note is that the cravings only last a very short time. If you do something else to distract yourself, like breath in fresh air a few times, then you will realise the craving is no longer there.

VAPING

Now that e-cigarettes are widely available, it is important to discuss the effects of this form of inhaling. With vaping, although you don't get all the additives that are in tobacco, there may still be some very negative effects.

As with conventional cigarettes, vaping is about having the feeling that you are breathing something in and breathing it out. As a result, both flavours and colours are added to make it more of a pleasant experience. The issue is that although the additives used in vapes are generally fine in the foods we eat, we do not know the effects of them when inhaled, and this could be very important.

There is already some indication that some flavours are not risk-free and, in fact, cause negative effects on functioning. Additionally, toxins such as formaldehyde, heavy metals, arsenic, and other substances, such as those you may find in cleaning products, may be added and these are all carcinogenic, which means they can cause cancer.

In Australia there is no state where it is legal to have nicotine in vapes and definitely not without a prescription. Even so, you may still be getting nicotine, as it is still possible to purchase nicotine vape juice, even though they are not legal. Nicotine is a strong and addictive drug, and has serious health implications.

Vaping can cause lung irritation and airway issues. There is evidence from the USA that vaping is causing a rise in lung disease in younger people. Particularly, there is a disease called "popcorn lung". This disease causes your lungs to deteriorate, and you will not get the same function back again[166].

There is very little indication that vaping helps people to stop smoking cigarettes. Tobacco companies are just creating more of a market for cigarettes and marketing to younger and younger cohorts of children. The most recent statistics gathered indicate that the annualised prevalence of exclusive vaping, and dual use of tobacco and e-cigarettes has been trending upwards with a big increase from 2020 to 2023 among those under 35 years old.

Additionally, this cohort was examined in relation to age distribution for both vaping and smoking. It was found that of those under 25 years, 34% of those were vaping and 16% of them were smokers (this includes dual use).[167] These results appear to indicate a growing e-cigarette and smoking issue that the Australian government is apparently intending to address in the long term.

You do not need to breathe anything other than air to prove to yourself that you exist and are alive. It is a fact that you do matter and you do make a difference in your life and other people's lives. There is nothing to prove.

DRUGS

It is possible to overdose on both illegal drugs and many legal dugs, through taking too much of the drug, or mixing drugs and this can result in harmful effects, including death[168]. Illegal drugs are more readily available now than they used to be, as well as more affordable. This is no reason to use them, since many of them have addictive qualities and a tendency to ruin one's life.

Opioids, methamphetamines, and crack cocaine are particularly bad in this respect. You don't need mind-altering substances to enjoy yourself. Make your decision to be and remain drug-free, maintain your determination, and don't succumb to peer pressure. You will find that you have a much better life being drug-free than otherwise.

There are also psychedelic drugs such as psilocybin (magic mushrooms) and LSD (acid). The draw here is for more of a spiritual experience, but this is not always the effect. If you are interested in being well-informed about the effects of drugs then you can visit www.adf.org.au for a complete run down.

In recent years, medicinal cannabis has become available, and research into drugs including MDMA and psilocybin has begun to show benefits for depression and trauma. This is, however, in a situation where a controlled dose is administered in conjunction with therapy. This is when these drugs are safe and legal. Trials are occurring now in Australia. For more information see www.mindmedicineaustralia.org [169]

PRESCRIPTION DRUGS

There is an increasing addiction to over-the-counter painkillers and prescription drugs[170]. Because these are often opioids, it can be very difficult to wean yourself off them. However, it is worth the effort and attempt. In the first instance there may be a good reason why they are prescribed. They are not a long-term solution though, and it would be more helpful to use them only as a short-term solution for acute pain. Once addicted, the drugs act on the psychological need, and may not even be all that useful in reducing the physical pain. In this case, the effectiveness of the drug is reduced.

Prescription drug addiction can creep up on you, so it is worthwhile taking stock of your health now and then, and to review what you are taking and why. If you notice that you are ingesting a lot of tablets every day over a period of time, then you can take charge of your habit and do something about it.

If you have chronic pain then there are other options that could be tried, such as hypnosis. Attendance at a pain clinic may also be helpful. St Vincent's Hospital in Sydney also has an online chronic pain program[171].

One particularly bad prescription drug that has been abused in recent years is Fentanyl. There is a high death rate among users[172], as the actual amount of the drug that is being consumed is unknowable. It is a very powerful painkiller and should not be taken recreationally. Because there is such a high risk of overdose, it is best to stay away from this and any other painkiller generally used in hospitals or other medical settings. Additionally, any new kinds of illegal painkillers that are being synthetically manufactured and coming onto the market are likely to be mixed with other substances, or be dangerous in their effects and thus should not be taken recreationally.

As a general rule, the reason why any of the heavy-duty painkillers are available only by prescription is that they are quite dangerous for long-term use and are highly addictive.

There are other options for feeling better if you are living with chronic pain, so explore these, rather than going for a short-term fix that may cause you more problems over time. Revisit Chapter 2 for information regarding managing chronic pain.

In any situation where you have an injury of some kind that results in acute pain, whether back pain, or other kinds of pain, there are much better alternatives than seeking medication over the long term. Look towards long term drug free solutions. These may include attending physiotherapy, or seeking help from a chiropractor or osteopath. These modalities specifically address injury recovery, skeletal and muscle issues and represent the best management. Additionally, it would be more helpful in the long term to engage in body strengthening exercises to alleviate future problems.

PORNOGRAPHY

In relation to pornography, there is a great risk of altering your brain if you engage in watching porn heavily and there is the possibility of becoming addicted. However, there are ways to use it in a safe manner.

In general, a proportion of what porn provides is

part of sexual satisfaction that cannot be satisfied normally. For some people, this may be beneficial.

For the most part however, the important things to note about it are as follows.

Firstly, porn does not show reality. It is not real life and does not represent what average people actually like or how they are. Additionally, images and so on may be manipulated and be completely fake.

The question to ask yourself is:

Am I doing this because I cannot do something in real life?

It is important to use it in a conscious manner if you are using it and to be aware of what aspects may be totally unlike reality.

One consequence of regular porn use is that it can actually confuse your brain so that you seek novelty from the actual searching and clicking on images and so on.

For males, regular porn use may create a sense of body dysmorphia. What this means is that a sense of a feeling of personal inadequacy may be created particularly in relation to sex and penis size, so that you may find yourself unable to undress or change clothes in the presence of other men, such as in a change room.

The fact is that men in porn videos are usually at the extreme end of the penis size spectrum. There is a great and wide range of penis size over the total male population. However, the fact is that penis size just as many other variables in life when it comes to people and statistics, is expressed under a normal distribution curve. To explain this as a mathematical phenomenon, imagine a mathematical sine curve, with the horizontal line being the x axis and vertical being the y axis, and the sine curve being placed along the x axis. See image (find one). Drawing a line that dissects the curve in half would put 50% to the left of that line – which is actually the average line – and 50% to the right. Most men within the population would fall into the average range- 1 standard deviation away from that half way point. The average is 68%- which is 32% left of the line and 32% to the right. So, most men would fall into this area. Then as you go further away from the mean, to the right, you go larger, to the left, you go smaller. Most men in porn videos would be far to the right – that is, to the extreme size, that is actually quite or very rare. Certainly not something you come across very often.

NORMAL CURVE DISTRIBUTION

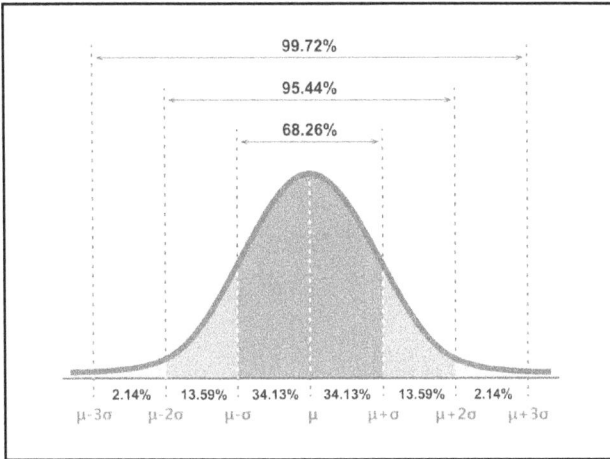

Thus, any assumptions you might get from watching porn may be completely wrong, and not just about how big your penis should be, but also about how other people like sex and how they should be treated.

How others should be treated is not what is depicted in porn videos and images. How others should be treated is with respect, courtesy and within the consent guidelines as discussed previously in Chapter 5. Porn does not depict reality at all. Watching porn can sabotage your relationships and get you started off with the wrong ideas.

If you remember back to the discussion in Chapter 3 on learning and mirror neurons, you will remember that mirror neurons enable us to imagine ourselves carrying out an observed action and understanding the intention or the why behind it. Essentially, what is happening is that it is also about identifying with whoever you are identifying with. But it is the mirror neurons helping this process. Thus, emotion will also be felt and this can intensify feelings. In this way, you may find that your feelings do not fit with reality, particularly relating to arousal in this case.

This is how your brain might become confused about what sex is supposed to be and be like. The answer is that reality is far better than becoming addicted to pornography. If you do feel that you are addicted to it, then the best thing to do is to find someone who can help you to create a more realistic idea of life and sex. Professional help is particularly indicated here.

Often it takes a number of close and personal relationships to sort out for yourself what close partnerships and relationships are about and how to be in one that is harmonious and equal. Treat others with respect and accept them as a human being who has the same rights as you: of being understood, being safe and able to make their own decisions about what they want to do is crucial. Take responsibility for your part in any relationship and consider any impact of your behaviour on any kind of partner.

GAMBLING

Where you have experienced watching betting odds and betting advertisements on TV, on the Internet, at football matches or anywhere else, then you are more likely to form the attitude that betting is ok and is a normal activity. While gambling is seemingly part of Australian culture, it is not necessarily a smart activity to engage in.

The consequences of betting on sports games can be the thin edge of the wedge. It can lead to a gambling addiction and gambling on a larger scale. It might be that you get yourself embroiled in gambling, and that it becomes difficult to stop, at which point it becomes an addiction. It is not too great a step from placing the occasional bet to becoming a problem gambler.

People who are problem gamblers usually hold a set of beliefs about gambling that ensure their continuation of the problem behaviour. They may believe:

- That winning is likely.
- That they can win back the money they have lost.

- That there are superstitions that will work to help them win.

However, none of these beliefs really hold up when looked at closely.

Whether it's the pokies, races, horses, sports games, scratchies or any form of gambling, the winners are not the punters. The winners are those who organise the betting and own the companies. The odds always stacked against you.

The betting agents win overall. You, as a punter, do not win. The chances, or odds, of winning are miniscule in comparison to the likelihood of losing. Just because you have fed a lot of money into a betting game doesn't mean the chances of winning now become any greater. This is because:

- For each game, or each bet, the odds are always the same and so the chances are new for each game.

- Superstitions do not actually work, whether it is playing a certain machine, choosing particular numbers, wearing a lucky hat or anything of that nature.

- The odds are still the same, and the chances are that you will lose.

Gambling is addictive for some people, and there are many problem gamblers who have ruined their lives through chasing their losses and not getting help for their problem. Gambling is, on one level, a means to escape reality by getting into a zone of excitement and hope. This does not have positive consequences. As with any addiction, if you become a problem gambler you can ruin your own life and also the lives of people you love.

Online gambling is big business— now more than ever. Although there is some regulation within Australia, including self-restriction for problem gamblers, there are still overseas platforms that can be accessed easily. What this means is that it comes down to self-regulation, and if this is a problem for you, then it is important to know where to get help.

More recently, overseas betting companies have upped their profits by urging people to bet with their mates. Other platforms outside Australia also offer different inducements. This is putting peer pressure to the test, by presenting gambling as a social bonding situation, rather than a lone loss situation. This means that you all lose together. It is not a winning situation. Why not just decide to do something together that is less destructive and more sustainable?

Speak up and seek agreement with your mates, and get support. There are government agencies and charities that offer gambling support. Don't allow guilt, shame, or any other emotions to cloud your decision or judgement. Try The 'Complete Men Foundation' for help[173].

You can stop yourself from going down the path of gambling addiction if you acknowledge and accept that a problem is developing, and get help from a counsellor or psychologist. There are also some specialist gambling services available. It is necessary to make the effort and ask for help, because it is extremely difficult to do it on your own. You don't need to do it by yourself. Get support.

While there are recommendations from a parliamentary committee to ban gambling advertising of all kinds in relation to sport, this move may or may not be a total ban[174]. However, this is unlikely to stop overseas online companies or other areas of gambling, so you will still need to be on your guard and educate yourself around all the previously mentioned problems involved.

GAMBLING SAFELY

Gambling can be a real waste of money, even if you are not psychologically addicted, or a problem gambler. It could be important to note those things that will help you to keep such a behaviour or practice to a safe level. Keeping the following points in mind may allow you to become more aware of what you are engaging in and how often. At the same time, you are more likely to stay in the safe zone.

- Make a firm decision on the amount of money you are setting as a limit when you know you are going to a gambling venue or similar. Do not go over this amount. For example, $20.

- Set this amount at the maximum you are willing to spend and the amount you are willing to lose. This is kissing goodbye to this amount of money.

- When you reach this actual spend, stop gambling.

- Whether you are in front or not. Just stop.

- Do not be sucked in by the bright lights, the excitement of others losing their money or (rarely) winning something.

- Be aware that the chances of winning lotto or any lottery is so miniscule that it is highly unlikely (eg. 1 in 2 million chance)

- Think about spending the money elsewhere where it can make more of a difference such as paying off debt, or going into savings for a big ticket item.

- If you do continue to buy lottery tickets and such, then only do so where you can definitely afford to do so. Mostly the winner is not you.

- All the same as above goes for poker machines and other games of chance.

- Set a limit, keep to that limit and then stop. Essentially, the lower the limit and the more realistic it is for your financial situation, the more money you will have at the end of the week or time period you are considering.

GAMING

Gaming can have some positive attributes, such as increasing one's skill, focus, increasing reaction times, and ability to concentrate generally. However, there are drawbacks if you become addicted to playing.

If you spend a great deal of time gaming, then you are not spending as much time on your life offline and in the real world. As a result, family relationships may suffer, on occasions communication with others in general may suffer, and if you only focus on gaming, then you may not be growing and developing as a person.

The key point here is perhaps the difference between being addicted and not. In immersing yourself in the gaming world, you do gain benefits such as social connections. Additionally, gaming is another way of story immersion and participating in that story world.

However, it is important that it does not become a substitute for everything. It may be important to set limits on your engagement at particular times in your development.

Your behaviour in the gaming world could be serving some kind of purpose for you, so think about what the secondary gain might be. If you are just spending huge amounts of time online gaming, then the question becomes what are you attempting to escape from? It is essentially somewhat similar to a gambling addiction.

Either you are trying to escape what your reality is in some way, or you are avoiding things you should look at and explore. Either way, asking for help may be important.

If you are a gamer, you could limit the amount of time you spend gaming through reducing the number of hours you engage in playing. Cut down to one or two hours a day, or a few times a week, so you'll be able to spend more time with friends and family. There would also be opportunities to find employment, discover other interests, and have some fun times with friends and family. The older you are the less time you should be spending gaming, because it is likely that the responsibilities you have will be greater, and you will be required to look after your own needs, as well as those of others in your life.

SEX

There is a difference between just being into sex and doing it a lot because of rampant hormones, and being addicted to doing it. While sex addiction can only be diagnosed and treated by a trained professional, some of the symptoms include [175]:

- Feeling that sexual behaviour is difficult to control.

- Feeling ashamed of such behaviour.

- Having difficulties with intimate relationships or with a known sexual partner.

- Having legal problems due to sexual behaviour.

- Hiding sexual behaviour from others.

- Having difficulties with work, school or social life due to sexual behaviour.

- Having a tendency to prefer strangers over known partners.

However, this does not mean that just because you have had a number of one-night stands that you are necessarily addicted to sex. There are several aspects that need to hold true before such a diagnosis can be given. If you suspect that you may have an addiction to sex then it would be worth your while doing some research and finding a psychologist who specialises in this area of addiction.

A SELF CHANGE PROGRAM TO FREE YOURSELF FROM YOUR ADDICTION

With addiction, there is often a physical component and a psychological component. Some substances have very difficult and potentially dangerous symptoms to manage when withdrawing. In this instance, do some research before you stop and also seek professional help. It may be that a drug addiction centre is the best place to withdraw from the drug in relation to the physical aspects. It is helpful to be armed with as much information as you need to start the process. Work out what you will do for the withdrawal symptoms—both the physical and psychological. Take care to use non-addictive substances to replace the addictive ones. Once you have worked out your strategies and have perhaps engaged in some counselling to help motivate you, you can start.

Drug and alcohol counsellors can provide Motivational Interviewing which actually does help to provide motivation. Monitor how you go. Are you successfully cutting down your use? While you are recovering from addiction, keep on rewarding yourself as you go through the day. Reward yourself verbally. Encourage yourself. After a few days, you could reward yourself by buying a small gift that has positive meaning for you. You could put the money you are saving towards a meal out, for example, or a movie night.

When overcoming addiction:

- Prepare – get information on withdrawal symptoms and how to manage them
- Explore the underlying reasons/issues on why you are self-medicating or engaging in this behaviour—a good therapist may be of use here
- Commit to the change
- Work out strategies you can use to reduce discomfort
- Where appropriate, avoid situations that may be triggers
- Have some counselling in this process
- Make a plan for management
- Monitor how you go and keep a record
- Put a reward system into place- unrelated to the addiction
- Usually, the more times you try to quit the more likely you are to succeed

- Use positive self-talk to encourage yourself
- Keep on visiting the reasons why you are quitting—keep renewing your commitment
- Reward yourself for positive movement
- Don't quit on quitting

SUMMARY

- Recognise and acknowledge that you have an addiction and then try to do something about alleviating the harmful effects.

- Take responsibility for your own change.

- Seek treatment from a trained professional, whether a psychologist or medical professional.

- Search and explore the underlying issue or root cause of this behaviour.

- Engage in stopping the addiction by yourself, if this is appropriate to your addiction. You would still need to do some research on how to go about this process and the best ways to do so.

- Work toward the goal of feeling more complete without having aspects of your life in difficulty.

- Ask for help when you need it.

- By taking these steps, you will be overcoming your problems and transforming your life.

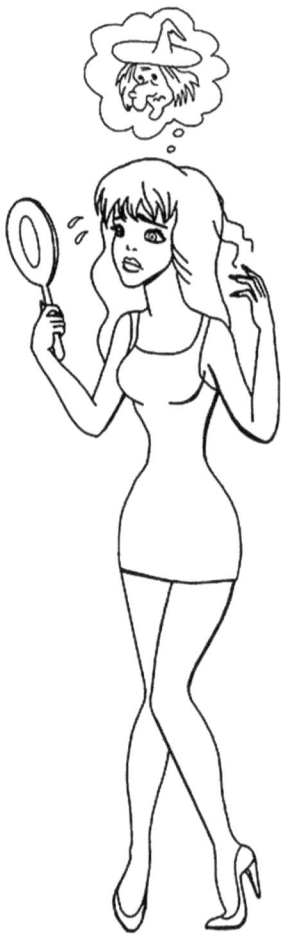

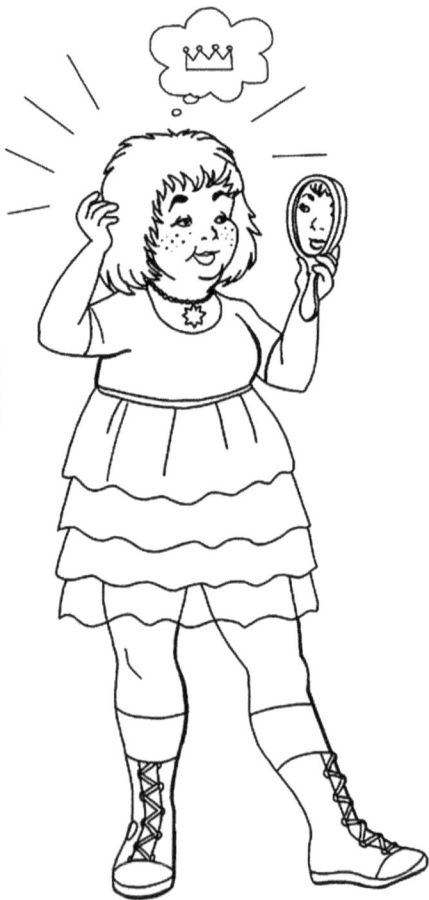

CHAPTER 12

SELF-ESTEEM

Self-esteem is your belief about you,
but self-love is how you feel about you.

When we are born, we are perfect little human beings, no matter what[176]. As we grow up, we get told how we are. We tell ourselves how we are.

There are pressures brought to bear on our perceptions of ourselves. If we get more positive feedback than negative feedback, we are likely to have a more positive perception of ourselves. If this is the case then your self-esteem—your belief about yourself—may be quite high.

On the other hand, if you get more negative feedback from others and you take that on board, then you are likely to have lower self-esteem. Sometimes, life circumstances mean that you interpret your world to mean something about you that may not be correct, and the things you tell yourself about you are more negative than positive.

Sometimes, positive role models can make positive impacts on self-esteem.

When May was young her mother always put her down, and so May believed she was useless. However, she had an aunt who was a role model for her and she was her saviour. May's aunt loved her and gave her unconditional supportive love. This helped May to believe in herself more. Further down the track, after May reached adulthood, she was able to draw on that belief in herself and breach some glass ceilings in her career.

If you don't really believe in yourself or have positive thoughts about yourself, then you are more likely to be passive in your relationships with others, as well as having lower self-esteem. You are also unlikely to accept compliments about how you look and how you are as a person. Everything is coloured by low self-esteem, and low self-love. If you tend to be passive, then the best way to overcome your issues and to develop yourself is to work on improving your self-esteem, and then work on improving assertiveness. You will find it easier to stand up for yourself and to be assertive after you feel better about yourself and believe that you deserve to be treated better. However, it is not just being passive that may indicate low self-esteem. You may have low self-esteem and also be aggressive in your communication style. It can go either way. The answer for both is to work on building your self-esteem, and self-love, and then work on assertiveness.

SITUATIONAL CONSEQUENCES

As we grow up, we gain a sense of self, and it's the interaction between the self and the world, including the feedback we get, that determines how we see ourselves, and how we feel about ourselves. If we get told lots of times that we are no good then that's what we will think about ourselves. This situation would lead to low self-esteem. Where we can master a number of skills then we might see ourselves as fairly competent in some things.

Self-esteem is, to some extent, attached to other self-beliefs, such as competence. Such core beliefs rely on an individual's capacity to be willing to try new things and to keep on trying until mastery occurs. Some people are more likely to do this than others. Those who tend to give up early may have low self-esteem. This may be the case when people are older than children. It is when children are young that they stick at things like walking and talking until they have mastered them. Once these things have been mastered, there are many other things to try.

EFFECTS ON SELF-ESTEEM

Praise helps self-esteem to grow, while criticism causes it to diminish. While it is not as cut and dried as this, this is a general rule that can be applied. However, it is not just a question of what others say, although this is very important. It is also what you say to yourself in your self-talk that has an impact. At some stage as we grow up, we take what others have said and we form an opinion about ourselves. Then we may tell ourselves negative things. In a sense, we take over others' roles. If you agree with the criticisms you have received, then you will criticise yourself. The younger you are when you receive these criticisms, the more likely you will be to accept them.

It does also depend on who is making the criticisms. Often, the closer the relationship, the more impact it will have. If you have a good reason to disbelieve the messages you receive, then you will not be as affected by them. The importance you place on the source of praise or criticism plays a role in whether you see it as deserved or not.

Some people tend to be innately more adventurous than others. There is also an innate tendency for extraversion or introversion[177]. These are connected. In general, the more timid and introverted people are, the more likely they will end up with lower self-esteem, because when they compare themselves with others, they find themselves lacking to some extent. Other factors, such as parental encouragement and praise, may help to override this.

The important aspect is that a number of factors feed into self-esteem, and it changes throughout one's life depending on circumstances and situations that occur.

One important factor as discussed is your self-talk. Another is external praise and compliments. Another factor is external criticism. If you are criticised over a period of time, then your self-talk may not be able to compensate and your self-esteem may go down as a result.

This process occurs in bullying. If you are in your teens when this happens it may be worse in its effect, since the peer group is especially important at this time. However, bullying at any age is the wrong thing to do to anyone. It is a very negative experience to be a victim of bullying and it can have dire consequences. The important thing to do is to tell people in a position of authority, such as parents, teachers, managers or employers. They may have some actions they can take to stop the bullying or alleviate it in some way.

IMPROVING SELF-TALK

Your self-talk can have a great impact on your self-esteem. If you say the right things to yourself, you can even improve your level of self-esteem. One way to improve self-esteem is by doing mirror work, as suggested by Louise Hay[178]. You look at yourself in a mirror, meet your eyes and say out loud to yourself, 'I love you (your name)'.

Say it as though you mean it, even if you don't believe it yet. Say it a number of times to get into the reality of it. Then you can find a good sentence that you can repeat to yourself as an affirmation. You need to repeat it at least twenty times a day. Out loud is good, but at least whisper it to yourself. The more you repeat it to yourself the more you can believe it, and your unconscious will be able to pick it up and run with it after a time. The first step is to do it consciously. It might take a month or so until it becomes easier to believe it and to think it, so stick with it. It might be a sentence such as:

'I love and approve of myself.'

'I love myself just as I am.'

You can start with something small, an affirmation that you can quite easily believe, and after a time you will internalise it. Once you have come to truly believe the affirmation, you can begin a new affirmation. Continue each affirmation for at least a month and notice the changes in your thinking over that time. Work up to saying that you love yourself.

Since you were a tiny baby, you deserved the love of others and you were perfect in every way. You have also deserved to love yourself since you were that tiny baby. This love is not arrogance, being "up yourself", or narcissistic. It is just the love that you give to yourself, as you would give love to another human being. It is a love that is kind and gentle, that is forgiving and encouraging. You need to do these things for yourself most of all. You are perfect as you are. It is important for you to accept yourself, no matter what you see as your faults. Faults are not real. They are socially engineered, and therefore they can go out of your reality and be forgotten. You are not just your body; you are more than your body. Similarly, you not your behaviour; you are more than your behaviour. You are not your thoughts; you are more than your thoughts. You are not your beliefs; you are more than your beliefs.

To some extent, self-love is a bit separate from self-esteem. Self-love is something you need to cultivate, so that you love yourself for who you are no matter what. Place the focus on your spirit/ soul, rather than your body. It might take a while to get your head around this, but perhaps trying to feel it may help. Loving yourself no matter what is extremely important. Self-love allows you to see yourself as already fulfilled in every way, just by existing, not having anything to prove, or need to do anything in order to receive that love. Loving yourself no matter what, no matter your behaviour, what you have done, what you have said, how you look, where you come from, where, how or what anything. Just in the moment, now, loving yourself.

In loving yourself:

- You accept yourself as you are, as you have been, as you will be.

- You only compare you now to you previously, with no comparisons to others.

- You understand that everyone is equal, it's just that some people have developed different skills than the skills you have developed, and have had different life circumstances than you.

- You recognise that you are unique and can make your own contributions to the world.

- You see yourself as an innately good person.

- You can continue to be the best you can be through flexibility and taking action to fulfil your purpose.

- You know that there is nothing to prove to others.

- You understand that just doing your best is enough—always.

- You are your own best friend and the only one who is always there for you.

EVOLUTION

You are as you are now, but "now" changes, and as time passes you will grow and become transformed into the future you. You will have experiences that you learn from. You are not static, but continually evolving. Just for now, forgive yourself for any mistakes you make and learn from them. Do things differently. There is no point in beating yourself up about them. Do something different next time. Accept yourself in your entirety and love yourself right now.

PATTERNS OF BEHAVIOUR

If your self-esteem or self-love is low, then a number of behavioural patterns may show themselves. You may be more likely to reject compliments by commenting that you don't deserve it or don't believe it or otherwise somehow putting the compliment down. Instead, try saying, 'thank you' and accepting the compliment.

You may also be more likely to become defensive easily and to take things personally when the other person may be just stating a fact about something that happened. If you find yourself doing this, then see if you can reduce your defensive stance and accept the facts. Perhaps you don't really need to justify yourself. The other person is probably not attacking you.

If you have low self-esteem, you could be more likely to pay attention to other people's needs, instead of your own. You may also play on this by acting the martyr. This may get you brownie points if others acknowledge your selflessness, but only *maybe*. If you do it too much people may get sick of it or end up taking you for granted. In the end, this game doesn't really stack up as being useful. And it's a game you shouldn't need to play.

Another possibility is that you become overwhelmed when the spotlight is on you. Self-consciousness may be an issue for you. This may be because you tend to be self-effacing and try to give others the credit when it's not necessarily warranted. If you give away your personal power like this then you could change your behaviour and allow yourself to see that you are worthwhile and powerful in your own right.

TURNING TO A MORE POSITIVE ASPECT

Improve your self-esteem and self-love, at least to a level of being able to accept compliments and not reject or deflect them. Hopefully, this level will also mean that you believe that you love yourself and accept yourself. If you are not at this level then work on it until you are. You might need to spend more time on your affirmations.

When you believe and accept the statement, 'I love and approve of myself as I am' then it should be easier to manage relationships with others. The first step is to improve the relationship you have with yourself. Once you have done this, relationships with others can be highlighted. When you know that you are ok then certain things follow:

- You understand that you deserve to be treated well

- You can share responsibilities and benefits equally with others where appropriate

- You can allow yourself to have some 'me time'

- You can allow your needs to be met

- You can ask others to help or contribute

- You can use the word 'I' in a sentence

- You are more able to stand up for yourself

This last point is why I recommended that you work on improving self-esteem before you work on improving assertiveness. If you do it the other way around, it won't work as easily and you may find that you get criticised for trying, and then you might go into a downward spiral. Two points here:

- You don't need to work on improving yourself until your self-esteem is at 100%. Even just starting to feel that you can accept yourself more than you did previously may be enough.

- Working on oneself is really a lifelong process. Although you may do this in stages and phases, it is definitely a lifelong practice. There is no end point.

POSITIVE SELF-ESTEEM

Where you have a built a reasonable level of self-esteem, then you are more likely to see yourself in a positive light in a number of areas. For example, you will be able to realistically assess your competence in performing a variety of different tasks. You will also be more realistic in your assessment of the standards you expect—for yourself and others—as well as your safety concerns and your ability to trust others.

You will also take a more realistic view when assessing situations as they arise in daily life. As your feelings about yourself improve, you will be much more willing to speak your mind when you are in a situation that calls for this. All of these things are core beliefs, and they include self-esteem. If your core beliefs are generally higher then you will be a lot better off in many circumstances[179].

You can complete a rating system of your core beliefs. If you do complete it both before you work on your self-esteem and afterwards, then you will get a good idea of where you are at and how far you have moved between each completion. Download the core beliefs questionnaire free at: https://www.dianahutchison.com/shop.

If you have relatively good self-esteem, whether through improving low self-esteem or as a starting point, then a number of things will apply:

- You are able to take compliments just by saying 'thank you'

- You are able to remain calm and to focus on the problem when another person asks you questions about an issue, rather than becoming defensive and taking it personally

- You are able to accept that you have needs, and that you'd like them to be met

- You are able to be assertive and take your needs, as well as others' needs, into account

- You are able to look after yourself by taking care of your own needs. If you are tired then you can say 'no' to an outing and go to bed early

- You can schedule self-care acts that will benefit you firstly, and others secondly

- You look after yourself so that you can take care of others and dependents better

- You are able to communicate your ideas to others in a manner that helps others to understand what you are saying.

- You do not need to play games to get one up on anyone else, and your communication is clear and direct

- You are able to go outside of your comfort zone and discover who you can become

- You are happy getting feedback from others, since it tells you how you are growing

- You are willing to grow in yourself and your skills—self-development doesn't scare you

- You are able to see yourself as loveable, so you do not have to prove anything to anyone

- You are able to have an equal relationship and negotiate agreements you make and keep them going

- Because you love yourself you expect good things to happen, instead of living in fear and not trusting others

- You can be realistic in your expectations of yourself and others
- As you love yourself, you can be more forgiving of yourself and also of others

Everyone is human and we all make mistakes. We can learn from our mistakes. Mistakes are, after all, just feedback.

Having at least a medium level of self-esteem can change your life in many ways. The major way is in your communication with people. Since we are social creatures, this can be a really huge change. It can touch all areas of your life for the better. The good news is that once you begin to really feel that you love yourself no matter what, then you will be more confident and feel more able to make positive changes in your life, and to take the actions you see are right for you.

Continuing to build your self-love and self-esteem will be worthwhile, because once you are even half way there, you start finding your life turning around.

SELF-ASSESSMENT

To some extent, self-esteem involves more of a value judgement than does self-love. What this means is that once you are able to just love yourself no matter what, then it will be easier to stop always being judgemental—of yourself and others. Everyone deserves love and acceptance. No matter what.

When looking at your life to get a sense of yourself and your self-esteem, count your family, friends, and education, and see how you are in relationships— both close and not so close. You can assess how you feel about yourself in reference to your relationships and your abilities in general. Self-esteem is the overall belief you have about yourself—just as you are.

While you may have self-confidence in your ability to do certain things and to behave in certain ways, being good at specific skills that may have particular importance to you also feeds into your self-esteem. However, if you have low self-esteem, you may discount your abilities and skills. These abilities and skills also feed into your feelings and beliefs about self-competence.

Once you have done this, set all of that aside and just take your awareness to your heart. Feel. How much do you love yourself? Score yourself for this out of 10, where 10 is 100%. Make a note of this rating and you can read the rest of this book and find out what you can do to create a higher rating for yourself.

Have a look at your life and relationships. What is the general feeling about these? Do you feel that they are generally positive or generally negative? How do they balance out? Do you feel nurtured in your relationships? Supported?

If you feel your friends are not supportive, or particular people are not supportive, then think about what could help this change. Is it your behaviour? Or do you think you could find different friends who may be more supportive? If there is someone who you feel is giving you more care, then perhaps see if you can spend more time with this person. Sometimes when we surround ourselves with people whom we like and who support us in our endeavours, then we can be lifted up and feel encouraged to do our best.

BODY IMAGE

Partly due to the prevalence of social media and influencers, and general marketing in the media, young people are more dissatisfied with their bodies than ever before. The point to know about you is that you are really who you are *inside*. You are not your body. However, the media seems to want you to feel worse about yourself so that they can take advantage of you by selling you things.

> If you do not already love yourself, or you have low self-esteem or self-love, then doing something to your face or body in any shape or form is not going to change how you feel inside.

You need to learn to love yourself first, before you decide to go ahead and do anything cosmetic to your body.

If you are getting Botox, for example, you are literally injecting your face with botulism, which is an extreme toxin. Equally, fillers and dissolving agents can cause severe problems. Changing your mind is not possible once you have had work done. A question to ask yourself is, 'Do people really like this look?' Ask them. The answer is probably going to be 'no'. Do you really want to look fake? And if you start having work done, where do you stop?

Influencers are not your best role models. They are often being paid for what they are presenting, and just because something suits them, this doesn't mean it is going to suit you. Nor does it mean that if you get what they have, that you will be suddenly be exactly the same as them or even be like them in any way at all.

Being physically beautiful does not make you happy. Physically beautiful people have problems too. The bottom line is that you just need to love yourself for who you are, no matter what.

Go your own way. You do not need to follow the mob. Be unique. As you are. You don't need to waste money on things that are essentially unimportant. Who you are inside is the most important thing— you are beautiful no matter what.

Although there are ways of improving self-love, self-worth, and self-esteem, such as doing the previously mentioned mirror work and affirmations, getting together with like-minded people can also be helpful. Other ways of changing your beliefs are to engage in NLP and Time Line Therapy™ with a qualified NLP practitioner, to find a good life coach or counsellor, or to attend a retreat, workshop or other event that may be of help. There are other therapies that may help change beliefs that you can research. You can seek out a qualified practitioner of your choice. Self-development groups can also be helpful.

SUMMARY

- Work on improving your self-esteem.

- Work on improving your self-love.

- Think well of yourself through affirmations and mirror work, by changing what you say to yourself every day, or by another method that works for you.

- Start loving yourself no matter what.

- Keep working towards achieve new feelings until you make the change.

- Think of improving your self-esteem as paving the way to working on improving assertiveness.

- Believe in yourself.

- Forgive yourself and be kind to yourself.

- By taking these steps, your self-esteem will improve.

- Through loving yourself, your life will change.

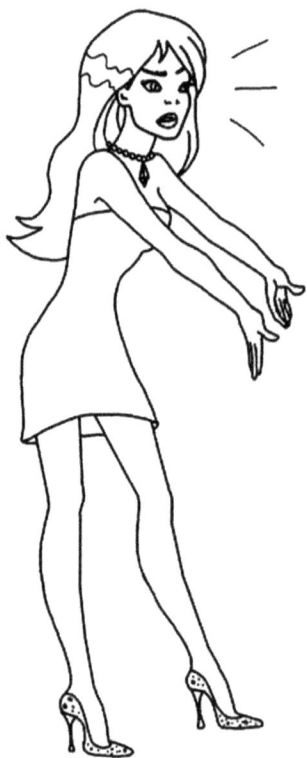

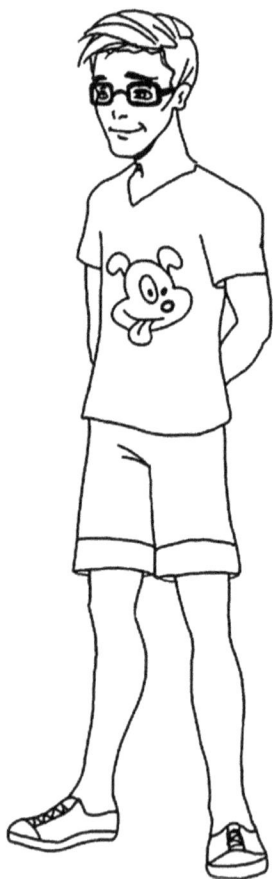

CHAPTER 13

ASSERTIVENESS

Do you understand how others see your communication style?

The best way to manage communication with others is to ensure it is clear and clean. When communication is clear and clean it is likely that boundaries are being respected: both for yourself and for others involved in the communication. Acting in an assertive manner treats the relationship as adult to adult, and respects boundaries. It takes into account your needs as well as other people's needs. Acting assertively is something you can practice and learn. It is a skill. If your self-esteem is low, work on increasing this as your first step, and when you have boosted your self-esteem to a reasonable level, you can work on increasing assertiveness.

COMMUNICATION

In any communication between two or more people, each person brings their own personality, attitudes, beliefs, values, and mindset. These may differ greatly. Additionally, there is the context of the communication and shared meanings of words, which may or may not be complete. There are, therefore, a number of ways in which a communication may be misunderstood. This is why it is important to use words that both of you understand, and to check with each other that the communication was interpreted correctly. People often make huge assumptions, and this fact can also make communication unclear. In the long run, the fewer assumptions you make and the more you clarify your communication, the more likely it will be that you get your message across.

Communication is coloured by our own beliefs, attitudes, and issues. There may be a way that we say something in a particular tone of voice, for example, because it is an issue for us. It might be a big issue or it might be a small issue, but nonetheless we may bring it out every time a specific context occurs. These sorts of circumstances may get in the way of communicating with another in a clear and clean fashion.

How you have an effect on the way you communicate may be an obvious thing. However, there are three styles of communicating that we are concerning ourselves with here. These are aggressive, assertive and passive.

The aggressive style is often threatening and demanding. The aggressor tells the recipient what to do, and may use a loud or confrontational tone of voice or hostile language. It puts the recipient into a defensive mode, and they may respond in a passive manner or meet the aggression with their own threats and demands. Aggressive communicators attempt to force their views and wants onto others.

Passive communicators generally agree to whatever is said and go along with whatever is arranged. Passive communicators do not stand up for themselves. They say 'yes' a lot, and can have low self-esteem and be generally self-effacing.

These ways of communicating disregard the other person's needs (aggressive) or one's own needs (passive). They are two extremes. On the other hand, if you are assertive then you are taking your needs and others' needs into account. You are standing up for yourself, but not blaming the other person. This is the ideal style of communication. When you have learned to be assertive instead of passive or aggressive then you will find that your relationships flourish—and as a bonus you get your needs met more often[180].

One point to note is that we all use all three of these styles at various times, depending on the situation and context. What often happens is that you prefer one style over the others—either in general or in certain situations. Check which style or styles you use most often at home, at school, at work, with friends, and so on.

AGGRESSIVE STYLE

It's important to recognize that assertiveness is not synonymous with aggression. While assertiveness involves expressing your needs, opinions, and boundaries in a direct and confident manner, aggression often involves forceful and hostile behaviour that disregards the rights and feelings of others. Sometimes individuals may mistakenly believe that they are being assertive when, in reality, their communication style comes across as aggressive. This can happen due to a lack of self-awareness or an inability to recognize the impact of their words and actions on others.

When someone communicates aggressively, they may use a demanding tone, criticize others, or impose their views without considering alternate perspectives. This approach can make others feel threatened or controlled, as if their ability to make choices or voice their opinions has been taken away. It creates a power dynamic where one person dominates and others feel disregarded, discounted, and disrespected.

If you find yourself consistently using an aggressive and belligerent communication style, it's important to reflect on why you feel the need to behave this way. Consider the impact your behaviour has on others and whether it aligns with your intentions and values. Developing self-awareness and empathy can help you understand how others perceive your actions and motivate you to change towards a more assertive style.

It's worth noting that different contexts may influence communication styles. For example, someone may be more aggressive (or passive) in a professional setting but assertive in their personal relationships, (or passive) or other ways around. However, striving for assertiveness in all situations is generally recommended. By adopting an assertive style consistently, you can foster healthier and more respectful interactions, promoting effective communication and positive relationships.

PASSIVE STYLE

Where you have a passive style of communication then you are acquiescing to whatever others are telling you to do, asking you to do, or expecting you to do. You are likely to put yourself last on any list, so that your needs are rarely met. You always give yourself the burnt chop. You may also have low self-esteem.

Women are more likely to be passive than men due to cultural expectations. It is possible that you are only passive in certain contexts, such as at work, or you may be passive in all situations. As you move through life, you may learn to become more assertive in a greater number of situations and across different settings.

ANGER MANAGEMENT

Anger problems may drive an aggressive communication style. If this is true for you, then you can get some help with how you manage your anger. A counsellor or psychologist can be useful here, as well as specific anger management programs.

Since we have seen that thoughts and emotions are linked together, if you become aware of your thoughts and beliefs—about yourself and others— and change these thoughts to be more realistic, then you can also change your responses.

AGGRESSIVE COMMUNICATION STYLE EXAMPLES

An aggressive communication style usually gives the relationship an unequal footing, since it relates to a parent/child relationship, and one where the power resides in the aggressor. An aggressive communication style puts things in the following terms:

'Do this for me' or just, 'Do this.'

'You must do it.'

'Do it or else.'

'You'll be docked if you do (or don't) do it.'

PASSIVE COMMUNICATION STYLE EXAMPLES

If someone is passive, they agree with almost everything that is requested of them or that they are told to do. They often give themselves the least or put themselves last. Again, it is a child/parent relationship, in as much as the other is seen to be better, more worthy and more valued, and to have more power.

A passive communication style puts things in the following terms:

'Yes, I can do that.'

'I'm used to doing that task, so I'll do it.'

'Yes, I'm happy to do anything.'

'Yes, ok.'

By working out when you are being aggressive and when you are being passive, you can then make a choice about whether you want to change your style and in which circumstances. There are going to be times when being passive is appropriate. However, if you are neglecting your own needs and wishes then it is important to become more assertive in the appropriate contexts. There may even be times when it is appropriate to speak in an aggressive style.

Overall, being assertive rather than aggressive is better and more appropriate in most situations. It is going to depend on your relationship to the other person or people, and the context of the situation. Sort out in your own mind how the communication makes you feel. Where you become angry or feel put upon, then perhaps you can change your style to become more assertive.

BEING ASSERTIVE

WHAT DOES AN ASSERTIVE COMMUNICATION STYLE LOOK LIKE?

Assertive communication takes your needs into account, as well as the needs of others involved in the interchange. It is adult-adult communication. In this style you are treating both yourself and others with respect, as equals and as adults. In this way, communication becomes cleaner and less manipulative. In the process of being assertive you are not blaming the other person.

When you are being assertive you are attacking the problem behaviour and *not* the person. This means that the other person is less likely to become defensive. One way to speak assertively is to use 'I' statements. Where you are asking your friend to stop putting you down, 'When I feel I am being criticised, I feel hurt and disappointed. What I'd like instead is to hear encouraging and supportive statements about me and what I can do. This will help me to feel more positive towards myself and you.'

In this example you are describing the behaviour and not accusing the other person. You are attacking the *specific* behaviour and you are owning the issue, since you are using an I statement. This makes it much easier for the other person to accept what you are saying and not become defensive or aggressive.

However, there are other ways of using words that will have the same outcome and create that distinction between the specific behaviour and the person themselves.

WHAT DOES AN ASSERTIVE COMMUNICATION STYLE FEEL LIKE?

There is also a distinction to be drawn between knowing how and being—information on what, why, when and how to be assertive and actually being able to put that into practice. Thus, being assertive. It may be that if you are guessing what being assertive is and you mirror from your own experience, then when you attempt to be assertive, the result may not be what you are hoping for.

Additionally, if you tend to be a people pleaser, then actually being assertive may feel like you are being aggressive.

Communication is not just the words that come out of your mouth, but includes: the tone of voice, the approach, body language, gestures, and the actual choice of words and your self-belief as a total package. So, it is important to get all of them right.

If you don't feel that you're allowed to ask for what you need or want, then your request may change into something you don't mean.

Exploring where your emotions come from can be enlightening too. Sometimes aggression may come from something being denied you. It may be that in a way you are denying yourself through your behaviour towards others. This may be an unconscious process.

What this means is that where you explore your own boundaries to become more aware of what you really need and want for yourself, you can then take steps to strengthen your boundaries. Then it will become easier to begin to ask for your needs to be met in a more assertive manner.

Resolution is more likely when using assertiveness than when using aggression.

Sentences that are useful to use when being assertive:

I feel_____

I want _____

What I would like is _____

Being assertive and the use of "I Statements" is not always going to work. It really depends on the other person and how they take it. If they are particularly aggressive then it might not work. If the other person is passive-aggressive then they might respond with something along the lines of, 'Well that's the way you feel', as though it is wrong for you to have those feelings.

What is important is to be honest, clear and direct, and attack the problem and not the person. Concentrate and focus on good alternatives and possible options in dealing with the situation. If you can think on your feet in the moment and keep on repeating the outcome you want then you may get somewhere. If this doesn't work then at least you tried, and you can try again with a different person or in a different situation.

It may be that you haven't yet found the right words or language that will work with a particular person. Experimentation may be helpful. Work and plan what you want to say before you are faced with a particular situation, and then you will be more prepared.

One thing that you can do to be assertive is to start saying "No" when you don't want to do something. There is no reason to say "yes" to things you don't want to do, be involved with or be associated with. Even if it feels strange and isn't your normal behaviour, you can start saying 'No' if that's what you want to do. No one who genuinely cares about you will think badly of you for doing so. They will accept it. People are able to choose, and saying 'No' is a choice. Accept that you have a choice and make the choice to say no if that's what you'd like to do.

Your world will not collapse because you say no. By saying no, you will be able to feel proud of yourself, and after saying it the first time, you will be amazed that it becomes a lot easier to keep on saying no to things you don't want to do.

Once you get into the habit of saying no when you mean it, you will feel more strength within yourself. It is a matter of setting boundaries. Paying attention to your needs and wants is an important part of this.

SOME COMMON PROBLEMS FOR PEOPLE PLEASERS

It is all very well to be amenable and want to please others, but saying yes to everyone is not necessarily going to get you where you want to be in life. You are likely to get to a stage where you resent others for constantly calling on your time and efforts. You can easily end up not having time for yourself, and your needs will be lost in providing for everyone around you. What this means is that you may end up losing a sense of yourself and who you are. When you realise you are at this point—if not before—you need to start saying no to some people and start meeting your own needs for a change.

To make a start on reducing your people pleasing habit, there are some things you can say that will help if you find saying 'No' too difficult at first.

You can instead say:

- I'll think about it
- Not right now, but maybe later
- I'll check my diary and get back to you
- I'm busy that day
- I'm not sure yet

You can come up with more ways of deferring giving a specific answer that will fit different situations. You could also say that you need some space, or that you need time to do something. Everyone needs their own space. It is also good to give others the space they need to do whatever they need to do.

Often, self-limiting beliefs help to drive our behaviours around our communication styles in various contexts. Such as:

- I'm not good at this
- I'm always doing things wrong
- I'm stupid

Change your language use around how you identify yourself.

Give yourself the opportunity to change, which may take some time and effort, but nothing is fixed in stone.

For more information about this, see my first book, *A Practical Guide for Self Change*

People may be able to be assertive in one area of life but not in another. If you needed to stand up for yourself against your siblings, you may find it quite easy to be assertive with your family.

However, this might not translate to your friends or your working environment. When you are with your friends it is important to set boundaries which you do not cross. For example, it's important to behave in ways that are responsible and within the law. You could set a boundary or rule for yourself that you won't drink more than four drinks or that you will be home by eleven o'clock at night if you have to get up for work the next morning.

ACTING ASSERTIVELY AT WORK

One area of life where it can be difficult to act assertively is at work. The expectation is that you will do what is requested of you or whatever you are told to do. As you are paid for your work, you are being compensated for this process. Some people think that this means that they can't object to anything. However, just because you are being paid doesn't mean that you can't stand up for yourself, within reason. It may well be important that your boss knows that you are snowed under and cannot do what they are asking of you in the time being suggested. It may also be of interest to your boss to know how well you have done with a project or job, especially if they don't always get kept in the loop.

At any work meetings it would also be important to speak up and put your viewpoint forward, particularly if you have a good idea that would be of benefit. All these situations, and many others, will require you to step up to the mark and say what you think. By being able to be assertive, it will mean that others will listen to you and take notice of what you say. Others will then make an assessment of you that is positive. So, take personality out of the equation, and just be remembered for what you say in an assertive manner.

In the example of being snowed under and being asked to do yet another task, you could say, 'I'm sorry but I'm snowed under right now. I can do it, but not this week. I'll be able to do it next week.'

If your boss insists on a deadline for this week, you could say, 'I need to negotiate which projects or tasks I leave until next week then. I cannot do it all this week. Will it be reasonable if I extend the deadlines for one of the other tasks I am currently working on?'

If you have a negative response here then you need to up it a notch and repeat what you said the first time. It may be helpful to go into detail about where you are up to with each task you are working on. Either negotiate which ones are left until later, or negotiate the time frame required. It will depend, to some extent, on the reasonableness of your boss. In any case, you will feel better if you say no and negotiate your way through it.

Where you are laden up with work and there is no way out of it, then there may be a co-worker who can help you. Where this is not an option, and you are being bullied as well, then it is important to find out your employer's policies on bullying and strategies on reporting this behaviour.

BULLYING

Workplace bullying often occurs over time and includes being spoken to aggressively, being called names—either to your face or behind your back, being belittled in front of work colleagues, being harassed, or being made fun of. The results of these behaviours create feelings of anger, upset, embarrassment, shame and a variety of other negative emotions, and may make you fearful of going to work and being at work. You may hate the situation but feel trapped.

Each workplace is required to have a bullying policy and a means of reporting it. If you are experiencing workplace bullying, then don't just take it lying down. You need to stand up and do something about it. Report it. See the Fair Work Ombudsman and/or contact your trade union for information and help with workplace bullying.

PASSIVE-AGGRESSION

Apart from passive, aggressive, and assertive communication styles, there is also the possibility that some people may be passive-aggressive. This occurs when a person appears to be agreeing with you or supporting you, but they are actually undermining you. For instance, an employer might agree that you can work on a certain project and then make it so difficult that you can't do it properly. This may involve them saying things such as, 'Yes, I'd love you to be part of the team working on the proposal for the new account. I'll give you the figures so you can write everything up.' And then, 'Oh, I'm much too busy to find those figures until next week.' Or a person may appear to give you a compliment, but when you analyse it, they have actually insulted you. For example, 'I really like your shoes. It must be difficult to find something that looks good when you have such wide feet.'

TOTALLY ASSERTIVE

If you are practising being assertive, then you need to get the whole package right. It is not just about the words themselves but also how you say them, your body language, tone of voice and so on[181].

Eye contact – practise looking the other person in the eyes to show sincerity

Body posture – it's best to face the person, sit or stand at an appropriate distance, and lean slightly towards them with your head erect

Gestures – gestures add extra emphasis. Suitable facial expressions show interest

Voice tone and volume – a level, well-modulated voice is convincing without being intimidating. No whispering or shouting.

Timing – sometimes it might be more appropriate to see the person privately

Content – it is the interpretation of the words by the listener that will determine the response

There is no hard and fast rule to omit the pronoun 'you'. It is, however, important to reduce the blaming aspect, so that you avoid saying things such as, 'You stopped me from leaving work on time last Friday, so I missed my doctor's appointment.' Or 'You made me burn the dinner.' If it is a positive statement then it is fine to use 'you'. Even in other circumstances it might be the only option to make sense of the sentence.

WHAT TO DO WHEN...

When you feel that people are behaving aggressively towards you, it may be best to ignore such behaviour. When you and the other person have both calmed down, then it may be appropriate to address the behaviour assertively. Initially, it is a good idea to delay your reaction and utilise positive self-talk, such as, 'Why should I let someone else's behaviour affect me?' and, 'Stay calm'.

___

It is helpful to rehearse future situations in your head or in real life, with a friend or in front of the mirror, for example. Work out what you want to say and how to say it, and practice your tone of voice and firmness. Then it will be a lot easier to get it right at the time you need to say it. The more you actually carry out being assertive in various situations, the better you will be at doing it. Really, practice makes perfect.

Assertion involves expressing appropriate feelings. Deciding whether an action is appropriate or not is a social judgement. However, it is best to implement the minimal effective response when it comes to feelings such as hurt or annoyance. For example, you might say to a waiter, 'I believe you have made an error in the bill. Would you mind checking it again?' In such circumstances don't assume that the mistake was deliberate. Don't, in fact, assume anything[182].

Being assertive is a good move. It helps you feel equal to others, and means that you are looking after yourself and other people's needs. When you are assertive, communication is clean and respectful. Others will also respect you when you are assertive. They will take notice of you and your requests. You will find that you make a difference to your own life. This means that your self-esteem may also improve.

Your self-beliefs are likely to increase in the area of competence as well. Overall, it is definitely worthwhile to work on becoming more assertive.

SUMMARY

- Work out your usual communication style, and work on becoming assertive in more situations where appropriate.

- Work on improving assertiveness one step at a time. There is no rush.

- Ensure you 'pick your fights': so that you choose the people, situations and events you know will be right for you.

- Ensure you use a calm and measured tone of voice and make requests rather than demands, whether you are an aggressive communicator, or otherwise.

- Start saying no in situations that are not too difficult for you, if you are a passive communicator, then move on to saying no more often, until you are used to saying no.

- Start speaking up and using I statements. Let others know what you really want.

- See yourself as equal to others and require your own needs to be met in realistic ways.

- Make your communication clean, clear and concise.

By taking these steps, you can become confident and assertive in your communication, and recognise yourself as being equal to others.

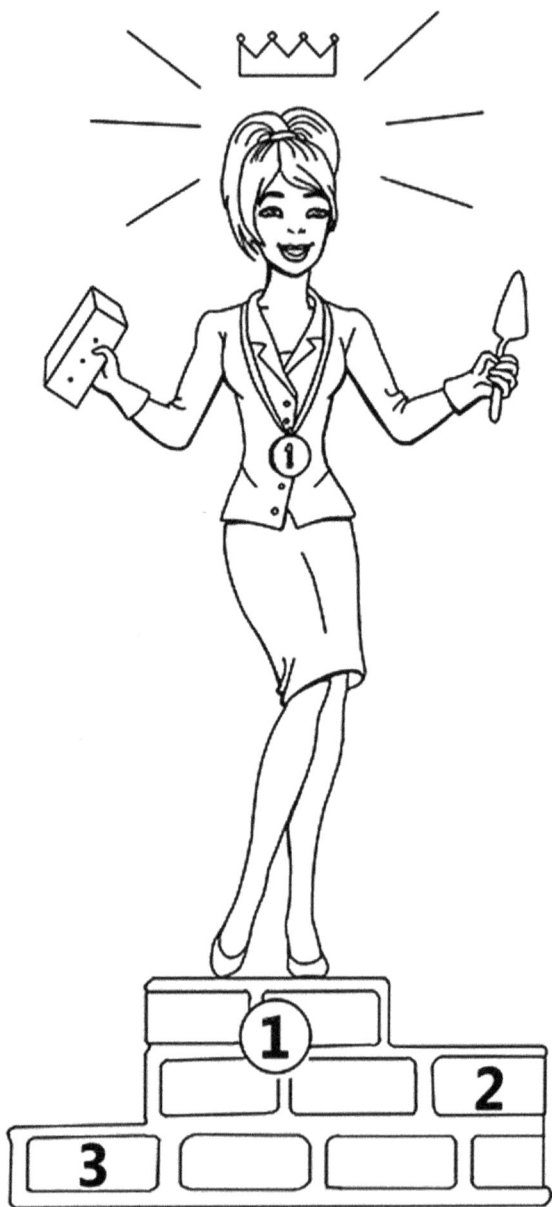

CHAPTER 14

PERSONAL GROWTH

If you consciously engage in personal development, the sky is the limit!

Personal growth is a good thing. When we change, especially when we do this consciously, then this is personal growth. If you have increased your self-esteem and become more assertive, these are aspects of personal growth.

Becoming more aware of your thoughts, feelings, and behaviour is personal growth. Change is a constant in our lives. It is much better if you help to drive that change by becoming a better person, dealing with your issues, and becoming more whole and complete. You will then become happier, and have the ability to make others happy too.

The first step to personal growth is to become aware that you *can* change yourself. Taking responsibility for actioning the change means that you take charge, with the understanding that only you can do it. It is important to work out what needs to change. Is it your self-esteem, assertiveness, or something else, such as how you relate to others? For a more detailed look at self-awareness and goal setting, see my book *A Practical Guide for Self Change*[183].

A couple of points to start with are to recognise that change occurs in the present moment, and it is better to spend the majority of your time in the present, rather than thinking about the past or worrying about the future. If you can do this then you will find many benefits, including increasing your happiness.

OUT OF YOUR COMFORT ZONE

At a particular moment in time, we may have personal boundaries we don't cross. Boundaries are good to have, especially when it comes to personal behaviour in relation to others. You can also have boundaries in relation to other people's behaviour towards you[184].

Boundaries for behaviour are different to those limitations you place on yourself to stay within your comfort zone. You can ask yourself what will stretch you in a positive sense, so that you can increase your comfort zone of skills, behaviours, or ways of being. What will cause you to grow? You could choose to do nothing and just let life throw you situations that you might grow from, or you could take the initiative and take conscious action. You might do a short course to improve your career options, or a leisure course such as pottery, learning a new language, or craftwork. Not only will you learn a new skill, but you will make new pathways in your brain. This is a good thing.

LEARNING MORE

If you decide to do a university course, investigate the career options that could eventuate. It is important that you are interested in the field of study. If you aren't interested and can't see yourself working in that field, what would be the point of completing a degree? It's also helpful to have some talent or skill in something that is involved in the course, whether it is maths, science, or the arts.

OTHER STRETCHES

If you are not interested in attending a course of some description, then work out what you want to do as an alternative. What would stretch you just enough to reach new heights?

If you recognise that you have some issues that need addressing before you can make a clear decision, then you could consider counselling with a psychologist or counsellor. You could also consider seeing an NLP practitioner. There are NLP techniques and Time Line Therapy™ techniques that are tailor-made for personal growth. Decide what you want to work on and make an informed choice regarding your practitioner. Make sure you ask questions about their qualifications, whether they are supervised or have peer supervision, and also ask questions about their philosophy of working with you. You will be able to tell from their answers whether they could be a good fit for you. Spending money on your personal growth sessions will be a good investment, and you are worth it. We don't spend nearly as much as we should on our inner wellbeing, and doing so will be worth it in the long run. Additionally, it may even be worth it in the short-term, since your feeling of wellbeing is likely to increase once you have addressed the issues you want to address, and begun to make progress. Also see https://www.dianahutchison.com

Goal Setting

It is good personal policy to set goals. You can then begin to take action to achieve them. Goals need to be **SMART**. That is:

Specific

Measurable

Attractive

Realistic

Time Framed

The goal needs to be:

Specific, so that you know what you are working towards and can clearly recognise when you have reached it;

Measurable, so you can track your progress;

Attractive to you, so that you are motivated to reach it;

Realistic, so that you can actually achieve it; and

Time Framed, so that you can check your progress as you go and review your goal regularly. A time frame also helps you to take actions and steps towards reaching your goal, so that you will achieve it in the time frame you have given yourself. For more on goal setting, please see my first book in this series[185].

Goal theory now recognises that different goals need different approaches. Goals are divided into two kinds. These are performance goals and learning goals.

A performance goal is something that is fairly straightforward and can be measured directly in terms of output. A learning goal is something that you haven't done before, or don't know what the output will be. In this case, the only thing you can do is your best. The important aspect here is that you are trying out new behaviours and seeing what you can do, and eventually improving on your initial behaviours[186].

MAKING DECISIONS

When you have an important decision to make, it will be helpful to use the Decisional Balance, which you can download for free at www.dianahutchison. com/shop. To make a decision, you divide an A4 page into quarters. You then label the two columns as 'Change' and 'Not Change', and the two rows as 'Good' and 'Bad'. Once you have done this, you make a list in each box. The top left will list the good things about the change you are considering. The top right will list the good things about not changing. The bottom left will list the bad things about changing and the bottom right will list the bad things about not changing. The good things about changing are the things that are motivating you to make the change. The bad things about not changing are the things that you want to avoid—they are the motivators away from where you currently are. The good things about not changing are the things that are blocking you and consist of your secondary gains.

Once you have had a fair amount of time thinking about these four lists, go through and rate each item on each list, where ten is the most important. Once you have done this, look through the lists and you should be able to make a decision based on all this information. It is also important to think about your feelings about making the change, and what may eventuate. As we have seen, emotions colour all we do. Hopefully you have considered these aspects in your lists. Once you have completed this task, you will know that you have done what you can to take all the information at hand into account.

INTUITION

Everyone has intuition. The question is whether you take notice of it or not. Intuition is your gut feeling about a situation, although it can operate as a thought that comes into your mind already formed. It can be a bit difficult to work out the difference between a thought you had and your intuition. Hindsight can be good in this case, to get a sense of which it was. You can teach yourself how you receive intuitions and then you can start to pay attention to your intuition more often. Should you do so, you may find that things work out better and everything falls into place more easily.

How can you know if your intuition is telling you something?

Sometimes it feels as though a thought pops into your mind fully formed. It can also feel like a 'knowing'. It is certainly not happening when you are pondering over something and thinking it through, unless, in the process of doing so, you find a fully formed thought pops into your mind from left field. However, don't let your desire for something get confused with your intuition, since intuition is often desire-free. It doesn't operate all the time, but the more you listen to it, the more it will occur. The ideas that occur to you from your intuition are not silly ideas—they are more about keeping you safe, keeping your loved ones safe, and getting the best out of your life. It is a positive and life-affirming force that you can use to make good choices and to take positive actions that enhance your life and that of others.

KAREN'S STORY

When Karen was twenty-two, she got engaged to her long-term partner, Tom. They were already living together, so it was a natural step to take. Once they had decided to get married, Tom went overseas for six weeks. After a couple of weeks, Karen went over and met him in Geneva. It was apparent that he was a bit disappointed to see her. She had a thought that the relationship wasn't right, but didn't listen to herself. They came back from overseas, got married, and had three children. Even before the wedding, Karen knew that getting married was the wrong thing to do. However, she'd had such a difficult life up to that point that she wanted the stability and security of marriage, and fantasied about being part of a happy family. Although Karen wouldn't be without her children, the marriage was never a very happy one, and she often wonders how her life would have turned out if she had listened to her intuition.

OPTIMISM AND PESSIMISM

People differ in their expectations of the future. They have a tendency to be either optimistic or pessimistic. If you are optimistic then you see yourself and events in a generally positive light. If you are pessimistic then you see yourself and events in more negative terms. While the pessimist may be more of a realist in thinking, it is the optimist who wins on all fronts.

Martin Seligman[187] has shown that optimists have better health, better relationships, greater tenacity, and, as a result, are more successful than pessimists. If you have identified yourself as a pessimist, it is possible to train yourself to become more of an optimist. If you do this, then you will gain from having this positive stance.

Pessimists tend to blame the outcome of an event on global, permanent, and intrinsic (inside of oneself) factors. For instance, if a pessimist fails a test, they might tell themselves it's because they're stupid. On the other hand, an optimist would tell themselves that they didn't do enough work for the test, making the explanation specific, temporary, and extrinsic (outside of oneself).

You can practice optimism by explaining outcomes you achieve in terms of specific, temporary, and extrinsic factors. You may need to consciously engage in this for a time before you are able to think like an optimist automatically more often. It will also be helpful to use this style of explanation in terms of other's behaviours, by giving others the benefit you are now giving yourself. People will be happy with this situation, as they will feel supported. Overall, you will become more optimistic, but you may not change your tendency towards pessimism completely. However, a greater level of optimism is a lot better than none. You should find that your health improves, your resilience improves, and your ability to bounce back from setbacks also improves[188].

There is a theory in psychology called "Attribution Theory". What this discusses is how people attribute the causes of an external event. To some degree, this theory links with a person's style of optimism or pessimism, although not always in a significant way. It probably has more of a societal, situational, and contextual basis. Thus, societal biases, assumptions, prejudices, and expectations may play a role, as well as individual aspects. In terms of blame, again it is better if you can put the responsibility for whatever the event was or is onto external, specific, and temporary factors. This is especially helpful if other people are involved. However, the context will be important to consider along the way and, in some circumstances, by not assuming but giving others the benefit of the doubt, you may be able to feel less upset than you would otherwise.

INTEGRATION OF SELF

Dan Siegel[189] has an interesting theory about health and wellbeing. The theory has our mind as the central player. He talks specifically about mental and emotional health. In his model, integration is both the goal and desired present state. Human beings are complex systems, receiving input from outside themselves, and with the ability to self-organise.

Emotions may lead people to states of rigidity or chaos when dysfunction occurs. When impairment to emotional wellbeing occurs, the movement is away from the flow of integration to either rigidity or chaos. Siegel puts the flow of integration like a river between the two banks of rigidity and chaos. The river of integration is where harmony reigns, and it is in this space that people are able to be: flexible, adaptive, coherent, energised and stable.

Sometimes we might move towards rigidity and feel stuck, or we might move towards chaos and feel that life is unpredictable and out of control. Being in the flow (of the river of life) allows us to live moment-to-moment, taking things as they happen and letting life unfold.

According to Siegel, there are eight domains of integration. These are: the integration of consciousness; horizontal integration; vertical integration; memory integration; narrative integration; interpersonal integration; and temporal integration. Integration can become blocked as a result of developmental difficulties or other life experiences. Any of these domains can become blocked, and problems or issues may arise.

In this instance, the aim of life is to remain in the flow of the river. In allowing, accepting, and being in the moment, we can find ourselves more in the flow of life.

Another concept of his is that of "mindsight". It is mindsight that can help us get back to integration. Mindsight is a kind of self-awareness which involves observation, objectivity, and openness. This is a process can be done with the help of a psychologist or counsellor, if not by oneself. Sometimes it is difficult to separate out the steps needed and the processes that will take you back to integration without outside help. One way to do it alone is through engaging in mindfulness.

Mindfulness is a process that focuses attention on

moment-to-moment experience[190]. By changing the focus of your attention to the present moment on a regular basis, you may change your brain. In mindfulness, you are getting your brain to be active, and this trains your mind to become aware of awareness itself and to pay attention to your own intention. In this way, you become aware of being aware, and you are able to take a step back and observe yourself in the present moment in a non-judgemental manner.

This is quite similar to simple meditation, and paying attention to your breath in the present moment. However, often in mindfulness practice, there are options to do things like body-scanning as well. Mindfulness is really just being in the moment, and focusing on where you are right now.

To exercise mindfulness or meditation, close your eyes and focus on your breath. With your awareness on your breathing, breath in and breath out. If you become lost in a memory or thought, when you realise that this is happening, let that thought go and return the focus to your breathing. Just focus on being aware of being aware and being in the moment. Start off with five minutes daily and work up to ten minutes. The more you do it, the easier it gets. After some time, you will be more at peace with your world. Do it alone or find a class in your area.

POSITIVE PSYCHOLOGY

Since around 2002, Martin Seligman has been involved in devising and furthering his theory of positive psychology[191]. Although undergoing some changes, he now proposes that wellbeing theory is at the heart of positive psychology. Wellbeing has five measurable elements that contribute towards it. They are:

- Positive emotion – such as happiness

- Engagement – learning new things, and being in the flow

- Relationships – that are more positive than negative

- Meaning – that you attach to what you do

- Achievement – achieving things for the sake of it

If you have all these elements and they are positive rather than negative, then you are flourishing[192].

A number of exercises are suggested that will help to improve your wellbeing. Have a think and see if you would like to engage in any of the following exercises.

GRATITUDE GIFT

Remember someone who is still alive who did something or said something which changed your life in a positive direction. When we express gratitude to others, we strengthen our relationship with them. Your task is to contact this person and say that you would like to do something for them as a gift in return for what they did for you. Your gift might be to do some gardening, bake them a cake, take them shopping, or just buy them a present and give it to them. As part of your gift, tell them how what they did impacted your life in a positive way and what the outcome is. Then discuss this and your feelings for one another. Doing this will hopefully help you to feel happier.

WHAT WENT WELL

This one follows the idea of focusing on what you want, rather than on what you don't want. What we focus on is where our attention goes.

In this exercise, at the end of the day for at least a week, write down one (or more) positive thing that happened during the day. Also, write why it happened.

An example might be that you had a good conversation with a friend. The "why" might be because she is a kind and thoughtful person.

In the second week, write down two things that went well each day, and why.

In the third week find three things that went well each day, and why. You will find that you are looking for positive events more often and you'll be able to remember them better. Consequently, you will start to feel happier. Sometimes this can be a challenging exercise, because usually we are looking out for the negatives. However, you will find that persistence pays off.

The positive psychology exercises should help you to feel better, happier, and end up with a greater feeling of wellbeing. In our lives we tend to like to feel that we are moving forward rather than feeling stuck and not getting anywhere. These exercises should help you to feel you are getting somewhere. It doesn't necessarily matter where you are going, it just matters that you are in the process of moving forward. This feeling of moving forward is, in fact, growth.

Personal growth can be intentional or it might be incidental. As you grow, you change, and as the days pass you grow and change in a myriad of small ways, so that after a year you might notice the differences. It might be that you have decided to do something differently, or even a few things, or perhaps you feel differently about something or someone. It doesn't matter how small the change is, it is still a change, and it may be termed growth.

> It is one thing to know the best way to be, do, and think—and to know how to achieve these things.
>
> It is another thing entirely to embody that learning. That is, to put the knowledge into action and practice.

How we approach our life experiences is something to explore. If you see life as a challenge that you can meet and overcome, then this is a more optimistic approach than seeing life as a struggle to get through.

Our attitudes and beliefs about ourselves and what we see as our purpose helps us find the courage to learn from our challenges. It doesn't matter if we make mistakes. Everyone makes mistakes. We are human. What is important is that we learn from our mistakes and start taking new actions that will have better consequences. We can learn from every relationship, we can learn vicariously from others, we can learn from information we find, we can learn from books and anyone we meet. We just need to be open, willing to admit we do not always know everything (because that is impossible), and open to incorporating what we learn into our own experience.

Growth may occur simply through the act of living—particularly if you go along with it. Personal growth can be hurried up by engaging in activities such as learning new things, and this will mean that the graph of your personal growth will rise exponentially. This is positive for you. It is exciting to learn new things, and achieving this learning will, as we have seen in wellbeing theory, enhance your wellbeing.

Plan to engage in an activity every year that will stretch you to some degree, whether it stretches your skills, your mind, or your body in relation to becoming physically fitter. Of course, it is helpful to keep your risk down, so do what is safe.

Stretch yourself just a bit, so that you are increasing some capability that you have. Every time you increase your beliefs about your capacity to do something, your belief about you as a person improves too—or at least your belief about yourself as being competent improves. In this way, you are working on your beliefs about yourself as well as upgrading your skill set. The more you find out in your self-discovery journey, about yourself, the better. Finding out where your limits are is still self-discovery. You can become more self-aware by working on being present in the moment, just as Alice did.

ALICE'S STORY

After suffering concussion, Alice's doctor advised that to heal herself she needed to stop over-thinking.

She found it hard to understand this, and was told that she needed to be in the 'now'. This idea was completely foreign to her. She struggled for months, trying to understand the 'now' and to cease her thinking. She would constantly catch herself in mind chatter. She became frustrated by her actions, and would start yelling at herself to cease the activity in her mind. In addition, she started to observe her behaviour. She realised she couldn't admire the ocean without getting bored, but could easily get distracted by technology.

This is when her journey to understand the workings of the mind and the 'now' began. During her research, she came across a concept of giving 'no reality' to anything that caused agitation. The instruction was simple: all one needs to do is repeat, 'I am not giving this any reality'.

She immediately started trialling this on herself and her family. Each time she felt any annoyance, she would repeat, 'I am not giving this any reality'.

As she applied this practice, she realised she was calmer, and finally experiencing the 'now', rather than being reactive, which had only ever resulted in her either becoming lost in thought or caught in an argument.

Her family and friends now also apply the practice of telling themselves, 'I am not giving this any reality.'

SELF-DISCOVERY

Where there are limits to your skills in one direction, this does not rule out going in another direction. However, it is important to be realistic. Where you find you do not have any particular talent in sport, then explore things to do with your mind. Learn a language, or something else you have an interest in. If you like words and are good at English then perhaps you could put your mind to creating a story, or you could write a blog about something that interests you. Be creative!

In your journey of self-discovery, it might be easier to work on obvious things first. This means that if you have a self-esteem issue then work on this first, followed by assertiveness, followed by whatever other issue you have. Once you have worked through your issues, you can expand your horizons and work on improvement. Improve your relationships, then improve your skills and capabilities. Personal growth can be constant. It can be a constant source of happiness and achievement. Making you and your life better may be a lifelong goal, which you can continually achieve.

SELF-COMPASSION

When it comes to criticism, we are often the hardest on ourselves. We may tell ourselves off and beat ourselves up over things we have said, done or thought. Your self-talk is very important, and if a lot of it is negative then you are likely to have negative feelings about yourself a lot of the time. It is important to be self-compassionate. Extend the forgiveness and kindness you would give to a friend or family member to yourself. The kinder you can be to yourself, and the more positive self-talk you create, the better.

The Losada Ratio (the ratio of negative to positive verbalised statements) also holds for your self-talk. So be kind to yourself. Keep on improving your self-love, and being your own best friend. You can do this the best, because you know yourself more than anyone else. Connect with yourself more, and be in the present moment more often. Take care of yourself and aim to be of service to others in your life, because this more than anything will help you to find meaning and purpose in your life.

SUMMARY

- Set yourself a goal every year to engage in self-development. This will hasten the process of your growth as a good human being.

- You may see self-development including spiritual aspects, creativity, healing, and anything you feel will stretch your comfort zone and be of interest to you.

- Work on your issues first, followed by improving your life in other ways, whether working on communication and relationships or learning new things.

- You can improve your wellbeing through the suggested exercises and others you find of interest.

- Engage in reading books in your areas of interest and those you are curious to learn about.

- Engage in activities that expand your comfort zone and stretch you.

By taking these steps, you can be the best version of yourself year after year and in the process, you will be consciously creating the life you will love.

CONCLUSION

I hope that your main take-away from this book is that you are responsible for yourself and you are the one who is in charge of your life and the direction it takes. Other aspects that you have gleaned hopefully include that all areas of life require consideration, balance, and moderation. Without health, we are unable to meet our best potential and paying attention to your body and what it is telling you is important. Since we are social beings, the better your relationships and your boundaries are, the more you can have a sense of belonging and at the same time, a sense of agency within your life.

It is unnecessary to be like everyone else. It is necessary to become more self- aware, to grow and become the unique individual that you are, with your own set of talents, skills and ideas that you can bring forth over time and develop in the way you want in order to become the best version of you. In this way you make a difference in your life and in that of others.

At the intersection of each area of life is you. Your values, beliefs and interpretations of your world are crucial here. In order to be your true authentic self, and to be true to you. While this takes time to work out who you are, the more you see yourself in charge of you (your emotions, thoughts, behaviour), and thus able to effect change in your inner world and outer worlds, the earlier and easier it will be to begin living a life you'll love.

In life there are many beginnings and endings – change is constant. Because life is inherently uncertain, if you see yourself as a person who is learning, growing, evolving and constantly changing to become the best version of you, this will mean that you are at the centre. Making the best of changes that come from outside, and making informed decisions that resonate with your values, you will be able to initiate changes that build on where you are at any moment towards goals and outcomes that you feel are right for you.

All the best for your future, and with this process of self-discovery and creating the life you'll love.

Diana Hutchison

REFERENCES

CHAPTER 2

1   P.D. Gluckman. P Hofman. & M. A. Hanson (2005). The fetal, neonatal, and infant environments—the long-term consequences for disease risk. Early *Human Development*, Volume 81, Issue 1, January 2005, Pages 51-59

2   P.D. Gluckman. P Hofman. & M. A. Hanson (2005). The fetal, neonatal, and infant environments—the long-term consequences for disease risk. Early *Human Development*, Volume 81, Issue 1, January 2005, Pages 51-59

3   Mlodinow, L. (2022) *Emotional: The New Thinking About Feelings.* Penguin, Random House:UK.

4   Neuroscience News (2023) *Technologically assisted communication may impair brain development, Neuroscience News.* Available at: https://neurosciencenews.com/brain-development-tech-communication-22285/ (Accessed: January 22, 2023).

5   Naomi S. Baron Professor of Linguistics Emerita (2023) *How chatgpt robs students of motivation to write and think for themselves, The Conversation.* Available at: https://theconversation.com/how-chatgpt-robs-students-of-motivation-to-write-and-think-for-themselves-197875 (Accessed: January 22, 2023).

6   *Why young people's mental well-being is in such decline* (no date) *Psychology Today.* Sussex Publishers. Available at: https://www.psychologytoday.com/us/blog/human-flourishing/202208/the-decline-well-being-in-young-adults (Accessed: January 22, 2023).

7   Schluter, J. *et al.* (2020) *The gut microbiota is associated with immune cell dynamics in humans*, *Nature News*. Available at: https://www.nature.com/articles/s41586-020-2971-8 (Accessed: 22 July 2023).

8   Neuroscience News (2022) *Gut microbiome at the center of parkinson's disease pathogenesis*, *Neuroscience News*. Available at: https://neurosciencenews.com/gut-microbiome-parkinsons-21981/ (Accessed: January 6, 2023).

9   Neuroscience News (2022i) *Gut microbiome at the center of parkinson's disease pathogenesis*, *Neuroscience News*. Available at: https://neurosciencenews.com/gut-microbiome-parkinsons-21981/ (Accessed: 22 July 2023).

10   *Taking probiotics with antibiotics: Does it help the gut microbiome?* (no date) *Medical News Today*. MediLexicon International. Available at: https://www.medicalnewstoday.com/articles/probiotics-may-offset-gut-damage-caused-by-antibiotics (Accessed: January 20, 2023).

11   *7 foods that are linked with inflammation* (no date) *GoodRx*. GoodRx. Available at: https://www.goodrx.com/well-being/diet-nutrition/foods-that-cause-inflammation (Accessed: January 7, 2023).

12   Neuroscience News (2022e) *Diet can influence mood, behavior and more*, *Neuroscience News*. Available at: https://neurosciencenews.com/diet-mood-behavior-21304/ (Accessed: 22 July 2023).

13   *Vagus nerve* (no date) *Physiopedia*. Available at: https://www.physio-pedia.com/Vagus_Nerve (Accessed: January 16, 2023).

14   Seladi-Schulman, J. (2023) *Vagus nerve: Function, stimulation, and more*, *Healthline*. Available at: https://www.healthline.com/human-body-maps/vagus-nerve#anatomy-and-function (Accessed: 31 July 2023).

15   Bonaz, B., Bazin, T. and Pellissier, S. (2018) *The vagus nerve at the interface of the microbiota-gut-brain axis*, *Frontiers*.

Available at: https://www.frontiersin.org/articles/10.3389/fnins.2018.00049/full (Accessed: 31 July 2023).

16   Porges, S.W. (2009) *The polyvagal theory: New insights into adaptive reactions of the autonomic nervous system*, *Cleveland Clinic Journal of Medicine*. Available at: https://www.ccjm.org/content/76/4_suppl_2/S86.long (Accessed: 31 July 2023).

17   *Polyvagal theory-useful narrative but still just a theory* (no date) *Psychology Today*. Available at: https://www.psychologytoday.com/us/blog/women-who-stray/202209/polyvagal-theory-useful-narrative-still-just-theory#:~:text=Critics%20of%20PVT%20argue%20that,value%20as%20a%20scientific%20theory. (Accessed: 31 July 2023).

18   *Contact us* (no date) *Intestinal LABS*. Available at: https://www.intestinal.com.au/chewing-food (Accessed: 26 July 2023).

19   *Processed meat* (no date) *Physicians Committee for Responsible Medicine*. Available at: https://www.pcrm.org/good-nutrition/nutrition-information/processed-meat (Accessed: 28 June 2023).

20   *Ultra-processed foods linked to heart disease, cancer, and death, studies show* (no date) *Medical News Today*. MediLexicon International. Available at: https://www.medicalnewstoday.com/articles/ultra-processed-foods-linked-to-heart-disease-cancer-and-death-studies-show (Accessed: January 6, 2023).

21   Wikepedia, Veganism. https://en.wikipedia.org/wiki/Veganism Accessed online 7/6/18.

22   Jacka et al (2017) BMC Medicine. http://www.deakin.edu.au/about-deakin/media-releases/articles/world-first-trial-shows-improving-diet-can-treat-major-depression Accessed online 11/6/17

23   Salas-Salvado J, et al. Reduction in the Incidence of Type 2 Diabetes With the Mediterranean Diet: Results of the PREDIMED-Reus nutrition intervention randomized trial. *Diabetes Care*, 2011.

& Estruch R, et al. Effects of a Mediterranean-Style Diet on Cardiovascular Risk Factors. *Annals of Internal medicine*, 2006.

& Estruch R, et al. Primary Prevention of Cardiovascular Disease with a Mediterranean Diet. *The New England Journal of Medicine,* 2013.

24   CSIRO (2005) *The CSIRO total wellbeing diet*. Penguin Books. Australia.

25   The Healthy Eating Food Pyramid. Healthy Eating Pyramid - The Healthy Eating Hub Viewed online23/12/2022

Nutrition Australia.

26   Good Sleeping Habits at https://www.sleephealthfoundation. org.au/fact-sheets-a-z/187-good-sleep-habits.html

Accessed online 18/02/18

27   (2013)   http://www.earthcalm.com/having-trouble-sleeping-may-be-an-emf-health-effect Accessed online 19/6/17

28   https://www.activebeat.co/your-health/6-health-problems-associated-with-too-much-sleep/5/ Accessed online 30/3/18

29   *Risks from not getting enough sleep: Impaired performance* (2020) *Centers for Disease Control and Prevention.* Available at: https://www.cdc.gov/niosh/emres/longhourstraining/ impaired.html#:~:text=Being%20awake%20for%2017%20 hours,drunk%20driving%20level%20of%200.08.   (Accessed: 28 June 2023).

30   Heidi Moawad, M. (2020) *Teenage circadian rhythm, Neurology live*. Available at: https://www.neurologylive.com/ view/teenage-circadian-rhythm (Accessed: 05 July 2023).

31   Australian Government Department of Health and Aged Care (2022) *Factors that affect weight, Australian Government Department of Health and Aged Care*. Available at: https:// www.health.gov.au/topics/overweight-and-obesity/factors-that-affect-weight#:~:text=genetics,healthy%20food%20or%20 be%20active (Accessed: 28 June 2023).

32   Trust Me I'm a Doctor, SBS TV Channel, Australia, 2017.

33   Ask The Doctor TV program, channel 2, ABC Australia (30th May, 2017).

34   Tapsell, L.C. *et al.* (2014) *Weight loss effects from vegetable intake: A 12-month randomised controlled trial, Nature News.* Available at: https://www.nature.com/articles/ejcn201439 (Accessed: 04 August 2023).

35   Find A Practical Guide for Self Change at https://www.amazon. com/books/author/dianahutchison

36   The Truth About Fasting. SBS TV Program with Michael Moseley. 2016.

37   Min Wei, Sebastian Brandhorst, Mahshid Shelehchi, Hamed Mirzaei, Chia Wei Cheng, Julia Budniak, Susan Groshen, Wendy J. Mack, Esra Guen, Stefano Di Biase, Pinchas Cohen, Todd E. Morgan, Tanya Dorff, Kurt Hong, Andreas Michalsen, Alessandro Laviano, Valter D. Longo. **Fasting-mimicking diet and markers/risk factors for aging, diabetes, cancer, and cardiovascular disease**. *Science Translational Medicine*, 2017; 9 (377): eaai8700 DOI: 10.1126/scitranslmed.aai8700

38   Neuroscience News (2023) *Timing calorie intake synchronizes circadian rhythms across multiple systems, Neuroscience News.* Available at: https://neurosciencenews.com/time-restricted-eating-genetics-22164/ (Accessed: January 6, 2023).

39   Crowe, T. (2023) *Dietary supplements have few benefits for most people, Thinking Nutrition.* Available at: http://www. thinkingnutrition.com.au/dietary-supplements-benefits/ (Accessed: January 6, 2023).

40   *Revealed: Many common omega-3 fish oil supplements are 'rancid'* (2022) *The Guardian*. Guardian News and Media. Available at: https://www.theguardian.com/environment/2022/ jan/17/revealed-many-common-omega-3-fish-oil-supplements-are-rancid (Accessed: January 6, 2023).

41   Timesofindia.com (2022) *Combining vitamin supplements linked to increased cancer risk: Study, The Times of India.* Times of India. Available at: https://timesofindia.indiatimes.com/life-style/health-fitness/health-news/combining-vitamin-supplements-linked-to-increased-cancer-risk-study/photostory/93751582.cms (Accessed: January 6, 2023).

42   Author Scott Gavura *et al.* (2022) *Liver damage associate with turmeric ingestion, Science.* Available at: https://sciencebasedmedicine.org/liver-damage-associate-with-turmeric-ingestion/ (Accessed: January 6, 2023).

43   Cassandra Green. *Major Public Health Alert on the dangers of taking too many poppy seeds ...* (Nov 16, 2022). Available at: https://www.bodyandsoul.com.au/health/major-public-health-alert-on-the-dangers-of-taking-too-many-poppy-seeds-news-story/cb4fadab858f5a5b89a22262dae4bc25 (Accessed: January 6, 2023).

44   Department of Health & Human Services (2000) *Food allergy and intolerance, Better Health Channel.* Available at: https://www.betterhealth.vic.gov.au/health/conditionsandtreatments/food-allergy-and-intolerance (Accessed: 28 June 2023).

45   Neuroscience News (2022) *Repeated psychological stress is linked with irritable bowel syndrome-like symptoms, Neuroscience News.* Available at: https://neurosciencenews.com/ibs-chronic-stress-21788/ (Accessed: January 8, 2023).

46   TodayShow (2022) *A beginner's guide to the Mediterranean diet - what to eat and what to avoid, TODAY.com.* TODAY. Available at: https://www.today.com/health/diet-fitness/mediterranean-diet-rcna63362 (Accessed: January 7, 2023).

47   www.eatthis.com/foods-that-cause-inflammation

Accessed online 10/6/18

48   7 foods tha*t are linked with inflammation (no date) GoodRx.* GoodRx. Available at: https://www.goodrx.com/well-being/diet-nutrition/foods-that-cause-inflammation (Accessed: January 7, 2023).

49   www.health.havard.edu/staying-healthy/foods-that-fight-inflammation

      Accessed online 10/6/18

50   Dizpensa, J. (2014) *You are The Placebo: Making Your Mind Matter*. Hay House: USA

51   Rankin, L. (2013) *Mind Over Medicine: Scientific Proof That You Can Heal Yourself*. Hay House: USA.

52   Physical ac*tivity (no date) World Health O*rganization. World Health Organization. Available at: http://www.who.int/news-room/fact-sheets/detail/physical-activity (Accessed: January 8, 2023).

53   Mayo Clinic (2017) http://www.mayoclinic.org/healthy-lifestyle/fitness/in-depth/exercise/art-20048389

      Accessed online 11/6/17

54   TV program, Australia, Trust Me I'm a Doctor, SBS, 2017.

55   Park, J.H. *et al.* (2020) *Sedentary lifestyle: Overview of updated evidence of potential health risks*, *Korean journal of family medicine*. Available at: https://www.ncbi.nlm.nih.gov/pmc/articles/PMC7700832/ (Accessed: 06 August 2023).

56   Michael Moseley The Truth About Getting Fit. ABC TV Australia, 17/7/2018

57   Garatachea, N. *et al.* (2015) *Exercise attenuates the major hallmarks of aging*, *Rejuvenation research*. Available at: https://www.ncbi.nlm.nih.gov/pmc/articles/PMC4340807/ (Accessed: 28 June 2023).

58   Department of Health & Human Services (2000b) *Walking for good health*, *Better Health Channel*. Available at: https://www.betterhealth.vic.gov.au/health/healthyliving/walking-for-good-health (Accessed: 28 June 2023).

59   Department of Health & Human Services (2000b) *Walking for good health*, *Better Health Channel*. Available at: https://www.

betterhealth.vic.gov.au/health/healthyliving/walking-for-good-health (Accessed: 28 June 2023).

60   Garatachea, N. *et al.* (2015) *Exercise attenuates the major hallmarks of aging, Rejuvenation research.* Available at: https://www.ncbi.nlm.nih.gov/pmc/articles/PMC4340807/ (Accessed: 28 June 2023).

61   Neuroscience News (2022) *Over a billion young people are potentially at risk of hearing loss from headphones, earbuds, loud music venues, Neuroscience News.* Available at: https://neurosciencenews.com/earphone-hearing-loss-21856/ (Accessed: January 22, 2023).

CHAPTER 3

62   Neuroscience News (2022) *Parents talk more to toddlers who talk back, Neuroscience News.* Available at: https://neurosciencenews.com/toddler-language-development-21982/ (Accessed: January 8, 2023).

63   Corfield EC, Martin NG, Nyholt DR. (2017) Familiality and Heritability of Fatigue in an Australian Twin Sample. *Twin Res Hum Genet.* 2017 Jun;20(3):208-215.

64   Bowlby (1969) Attachment and Loss. Penguin:UK.

65   Meier, J.D. (no date) *Nature vs nurture?, Sources of Insight.* Available at: https://sourcesofinsight.com/nature-vs-nurture/#:~:text=In%20every%20study%20of%20its,your%20mother%20and%20your%20father.%E2%80%9D&text=The%20other%2050%20percent%20is%20not%20nurture%20by%20your%20parents. (Accessed: 26 July 2023).

66   Seligman, M.E.P. (1992) *Learned Optimism.* Random House: Australia.

67   Seligman, M.E.P. (1993) *What You Can Change..And What You Can't.* Ballentine:USA

68   Acharya, S. and Shukla, S. (2012) 'Mirror neurons: Enigma of the metaphysical modular brain', *Journal of Natural Science,*

Biology and Medicine, 3(2), p. 118. doi:10.4103/0976-9668.101878. (Accessed online 2/8/23)

69   Preston SD, de Waal FB. Empathy: Its ultimate and proximate bases. Behavioral Brain Science. 2002;25:1-72. Cited by Acharya, S. and Shukla, S. (2012) 'Mirror neurons: Enigma of the metaphysical modular brain', *Journal of Natural Science, Biology and Medicine*, 3(2), p. 118. doi:10.4103/0976-9668.101878. (Accessed online 2/8/23)

70   Gallese V, Keysers C, Rizzolatti G. A unifying view of the basis of social cognition. Trends in Cognition Science. 2004;8:396-403. Cited by Acharya, S. and Shukla, S. (2012) 'Mirror neurons: Enigma of the metaphysical modular brain', *Journal of Natural Science, Biology and Medicine*, 3(2), p. 118. doi:10.4103/0976-9668.101878. (Accessed online 2/8/23)

71   McKay, M. & Fanning, P. (1991) *Prisoners of Belief*. New Harbinger: USA

72   . Elliott, (1970) *The Eye of the Storm*. ABC:USA

https://en.wikipedia.org/wiki/Jane_Elliott#First_exercise_involving_eye_color_and_brown_collars

Accessed 12/6/17

CHAPTER 4

73   https://mic.com/articles/106764/why-it-s-better-to-have-4-amazing-friends-than-400-just-ok-ones#.1AMk8HRHG

Accessed online 15/7/2018

74   https://www.lifehacker.com.au/2018/03/this-is-how-many-friends-you-need-to-be-happy/

Accessed online 15/7/2018

75   http://www.thisisinsider.com/being-best-friends-with-spouse-benefits-2018-3

Accessed online 15/7/2018

76   Haupt, A. (2023) *Yes, single people can be happy and healthy,*

Time. Available at: https://time.com/6255111/single-people-happy-healthy/#:~:text=People%20become%20more%20satisfied%20with,satisfied%20with%20their%20solo%20lives. (Accessed: 05 July 2023).

77 . Bowlby (1969) Attachment and Loss. Penguin:UK.

78 Hughes, Dan (2013) *8 Keys to Building Your Best Relationships (8 Keys to Mental Health)*. WW Norton & Company: New York.

79 . Hughes, Dan (2013) *8 Keys to Building Your Best Relationships (8 Keys to Mental Health)*. WW Norton & Company: New York.

80 Seligman, M.E.P. (1993) *What You Can Change..And What You Can't*. Ballentine:USA

81 Jo Nash, P.D. (2022) *How to set healthy boundaries & build positive relationships*, *PositivePsychology.com*. Available at: https://positivepsychology.com/great-self-care-setting-healthy-boundaries/#relation (Accessed: January 8, 2023).

82 *Boundaries and Dysfunctional Family Systems* (2019) *MentalHelp.net*. Available at: https://www.mentalhelp.net/psychotherapy/boundaries-and-dysfunctional-family-systems/ (Accessed: January 8, 2023).

83 *Apa Dictionary of Psychology* (no date) *American Psychological Association*. Available at: https://dictionary.apa.org/enmeshment (Accessed: 26 July 2023).

84 *Boundaries and Dysfunctional Family Systems* (2019) *MentalHelp.net*. Available at: https://www.mentalhelp.net/psychotherapy/boundaries-and-dysfunctional-family-systems/ (Accessed: January 8, 2023).

85 Pattemore, C. (2021) *10 ways to build and preserve better boundaries*, *Psych Central*. Psych Central. Available at: https://psychcentral.com/lib/10-way-to-build-and-preserve-better-boundaries (Accessed: January 8, 2023).

86 All Pro Dad (2020) *10 ways to establish clear boundaries for children*, *All Pro Dad*. Available at: http://www.allprodad.com/10-ways-to-establish-clear-boundaries-for-children/ (Accessed: January 8, 2023).

87 *Circadian rhythms: What time is your brain at its cognitive peak?* (2022) *Big Think*. Available at: https://bigthink.com/neuropsych/circadian-rhythms-brain-cognitive-peak/ (Accessed: January 8, 2023).

88 Ellwood, B. (2022) *Boys and girls have different expectations about friendship, and these gender differences increase during adolescence*, *PsyPost*. Available at: https://www.psypost.org/2022/07/boys-and-girls-have-different-expectations-about-friendship-and-these-gender-differences-increase-during-adolescence-63492 (Accessed: January 7, 2023).

89 *Building healthy romantic relationships: Headspace* (no date) *headspace National Youth Mental Health Foundation*. Available at: https://headspace.org.au/explore-topics/for-young-people/healthy-romantic-relationships/ (Accessed: January 8, 2023).

90 Seligman, M. (2011) *Flourish*. Random House: Australia.

91 Hutchison, D.E. (2022) A Practical Guide for Self Change. Self Published. Available at www.amazon.com/books/author/dianahutchison

CHAPTER 5

92 Seligman, M.E.P. (1993) *What You Can Change..And What You Can't*. Ballentine:USA

93 Seligman, M.E.P. (1993) *What You Can Change..And What You Can't*. Ballentine:USA

94 *Helplines, telephone and online counselling services for children, young people and adults* (no date) *AIFS*. Available at: https://aifs.gov.au/resources/resource-sheets/helplines-telephone-and-online-counselling-services-children-young-people (Accessed: January 12, 2023).

Kids Helpline 1800 55 1800

Headspace: www.headspace.org.au

Lifeline: www.lifeline.org.au 13 11 14

Wesley Mission: www.wesleymission.org.au Mental Health 1300 924 522

For sexual assault, domestic and family violence: 1800 737 732

95 *Stis* (2022) *STI Guidelines Australia*. Available at: https://sti. guidelines.org.au/sexually-transmissible-infections/ (Accessed: 26 July 2023).

96 *Key populations in the Australian HIV epidemic* (no date) *HIV Management Guidelines*. Available at: https://hivmanagement. ashm.org.au/the-epidemiology-of-hiv-in-australia/key-populations-in-the-australian-hiv-epidemic/ (Accessed: 27 July 2023).

97 *Building healthy romantic relationships: Headspace* (no date) *headspace National Youth Mental Health Foundation*. Available at: https://headspace.org.au/explore-topics/for-young-people/ healthy-romantic-relationships/ (Accessed: January 12, 2023).

98 *Family, domestic and sexual violence* (no date) *Australian Institute of Health and Welfare*. Available at: https://www.aihw. gov.au/reports/domestic-violence/family-domestic-and-sexual-violence (Accessed: January 12, 2023).

99 Australian Institute of Criminology (2020) *The prevalence of domestic violence among women during the COVID-19 pandemic domestic violence against women during covid-19 in Australia*, *Australian Institute of Criminology*. Available at: https://www. aic.gov.au/publications/sb/sb28#:~:text=Almost%20six%20 percent%20(5.8%25),escalation%20of%20violence%20 and%20abuse. (Accessed: 27 July 2023).

100 Frayne, A. (2021) *Domestic coercive control could soon be criminal in Australia - family law - australia, Domestic coercive control could soon be criminal in Australia - Family Law - Australia*. Available at: https://www.mondaq.com/australia/ family-law/1108818/domestic-coercive-control-could-soon-be-criminal-in-australia#:~:text=Other%20jurisdictions%20 have%20introduced%20offences,and%20economic%20abuse-%20in%202005. (Accessed: 27 July 2023).

101 *Toora Women Inc..* (2023) *Toora Women Inc.* Available at: https://www.toora.org.au/ (Accessed: 27 July 2023).

102 Neuroscience News (2022m) *How trauma changes the brain*, *Neuroscience News*. Available at: https://neurosciencenews. com/?p=88765 (Accessed: 05 July 2023).

CHAPTER 7

103 Cairns, Julie Ann (2015) *The Abundance Code: How to Bust the 7 Money Myths for a Rich Life Now.* Hay House Inc.:US

104 Castrillon, C. (2023) *5 ways to go from a scarcity to abundance mindset*, *Forbes*. Available at: https://www.forbes.com/sites/carolinecastrillon/2020/07/12/5-ways-to-go-from-a-scarcity-to-abundance-mindset/?sh=612eb2ca1197 (Accessed: 29 July 2023).

105 Kiyosaki, R.T., (2017). *Rich dad, poor dad*, (2nd Ed) Scottsdale, AZ: Plata Publishing.

106 Pape, Scott (2017) *The Barefoot Investor:The only money guide you'll ever need.* Barefoot Investor Management Pty Ltd. Wiley & Sons. Melbourne, Australia.

107 https://www.moneysmart.gov.au *Home* (no date) *Home - Moneysmart.gov.au*. Available at: https://moneysmart.gov.au/ (Accessed: January 12, 2023).

108 Pape, Scott (2017) *The Barefoot Investor:The only money guide you'll ever need.* Barefoot Investor Management Pty Ltd. Wiley & Sons. Melbourne, Australia.

109 Pape, S. (2022) *Barefoot Kids: Your epic money adventure*. Melbourne, VIC: Barefoot Publishing.

110 Hutchison, D.E. (2022) A Practical Guide for Self Change. Self Published. Available at www.amazon.com/books/author/dianahutchison

111 In Australia, one such ethical microfinance company is Good Shepherd Microfinance

112 https://www.moneysmart.gov.au *Home* (no date) *Home - Moneysmart.gov.au*. Available at: https://moneysmart.gov.au/ (Accessed: January 12, 2023).

113 *Protect yourself from scams - moneysmart* (no date). Available at: https://static.moneysmart.gov.au/files/publications/protect-yourself-from-scams.pdf (Accessed: January 12, 2023).

114 Australian Competition and Consumer Commission (2023) *Home: Scamwatch, Australian Competition and Consumer Commission*. Australian Competition and Consumer Commission. Available at: https://www.scamwatch.gov.au/ (Accessed: January 12, 2023).

CHAPTER 8

115 Holland, J. L. (1988) *Self Directed Search*. Edited by Jan Lokan. Australian Edition. Adapted from the American SDS Published by Psychological Assessment Resources with permission. ACER.

116 *Discover your passion: Self-directed search* (2022) *SDS Development*. Available at: https://self-directed-search.com/ (Accessed: January 13, 2023).

117 http://www.abc.net.au/news/2017-11-14/communication-interpersonal-skills-could-trump-stem-at-work/9148528

     ABC article about future jobs. Accessed 14/11/17

118 Climate Council (2019) *Australia among worst emitters in the world, Climate Council*. Available at: https://www.climatecouncil.org.au/australia-among-worst-emitters-world/?atb=DSA01b&gclid=Cj0KCQiA_P6dBhD1ARIsAAGI7HCoE8NSGxxQUubP5VOwvaNO0zKcbGTsCULyMvm1GWVZThZS0kmwIzoaAqNrEALw_wcB (Accessed: January 13, 2023).

119 (no date) *Welcome to the Fair Work Ombudsman website*. Available at: https://www.fairwork.gov.au/ (Accessed: January 13, 2023).

120 *Pay guides* (no date) *Pay guides - Fair Work Ombudsman*.

Available at: https://www.fairwork.gov.au/pay-and-wages/minimum-wages/pay-guides (Accessed: January 13, 2023).

121 Neuroscience News (2022) *Higher sense of purpose in life may be linked to lower mortality risk*, *Neuroscience News*. Available at: https://neurosciencenews.com/mortality-sense-purpose-21864/ (Accessed: January 13, 2023).

CHAPTER 9

122 *Damasio, A. R. (1994). descartes' error: Emotion, reason and the human ...* (no date). Available at: https://www.jstor.org/stable/2653504 (Accessed: January 13, 2023).

123 Mlodinow, Leonard (2022) *Emotional: The New Thinking About Feelings*. Penguin Random House, UK.

124 *Understanding violence* (no date) *Workplace Equality and Respect | Our Watch*. Available at: https://workplace.ourwatch.org.au/understanding-violence-and-sexual-harassment/ (Accessed: January 13, 2023).

125 Gendlin, E.T. (1981) *Focusing.* Bantam Books:USA

126 Lorelie, C. (2022) *Talking to strangers helps you feel happier & more connected*, *Medium*. getHapi. Available at: https://medium.com/gethapi/talking-to-strangers-helps-you-feel-happier-more-connected-b0ab0554da18 (Accessed: January 13, 2023).

127 Chai, C. *et al.* (no date) *Loneliness: Causes, coping with it, and getting help*, *EverydayHealth.com*. Available at: https://www.everydayhealth.com/loneliness/ (Accessed: January 13, 2023).

CHAPTER 10

128 *Chronic disease center (NCCDPHP)* (2023) *Centers for Disease Control and Prevention*. Available at: https://www.cdc.gov/chronicdisease/index.htm (Accessed: 30 July 2023).

129 *Mental Health Services in Australia: Mental health: Prevalence and impact* (no date) *Australian Institute of Health and Welfare*. Available at: https://www.aihw.gov.au/reports/mental-health-services/mental-health#Common (Accessed: 30 July 2023).

130 Butler, A. C., Chapman, J. E., Forman, E. M., & Beck, A. T. (2006). The empirical status of cognitive-behavioural therapy: A review of meta analyses. *Clinical Psychology Review*, 26, 17-31.

131 University, D. (no date) *World-first trial shows improving diet can treat major depression, Deakin University*. Available at: https://www.deakin.edu.au/about-deakin/news-and-media-releases/articles/world-first-trial-shows-improving-diet-can-treat-major-depression (Accessed: January 13, 2023).

132 Worden, J. William (2018) (5th Ed) *Grief Counseling and Grief Therapy: A Handbook for the Mental Health Practitioner.* Springer Publishing Company: USA.

133 Worden, J. William (2018) (5th Ed) *Grief Counseling and Grief Therapy: A Handbook for the Mental Health Practitioner.* Springer Publishing Company: USA.

134 APS (2017) https://www.psychology.org.au/psychologyweek/survey/results-fomo/ Accessed online 19/6/17

135 *Teens suffer highest rates of Fomo* (no date) *Teens suffer highest rates of FOMO | APS*. Available at: https://psychology.org.au/news/media_releases/8nov2015-fomo (Accessed: January 15, 2023).

136 White, M.P. *et al.* (2019) *Spending at least 120 minutes a week in nature is associated with good health and Wellbeing, Nature News*. Available at: https://www.nature.com/articles/s41598-019-44097-3 (Accessed: 30 July 2023).

137 *Home - eating disorders victoria - services and support for those affected.* (2022) *Eating Disorders Victoria*. Available at: https://www.eatingdisorders.org.au/ (Accessed: January 15, 2023).

138 *Anorexia nervosa* (2021) *Butterfly Foundation*. Available at: https://butterfly.org.au/eating-disorders/eating-disorders-explained/anorexia-nervosa/ (Accessed: 30 July 2023).

139 Miller, Caroline A (2014) *My Name is Caroline* (2nd Ed.) Cogent Publishing:USA

140 *Avoidant restrictive food intake disorder (ARFID)* (2018) *National Eating Disorders Association.* Available at: https://www.nationaleatingdisorders.org/learn/by-eating-disorder/arfid (Accessed: January 15, 2023).

141 *Avoidant restrictive food intake disorder (ARFID)* (2018) *National Eating Disorders Association.* Available at: https://www.nationaleatingdisorders.org/learn/by-eating-disorder/arfid (Accessed: January 15, 2023).

142 *Home - eating disorders victoria - services and support for those affected.* (2022) *Eating Disorders Victoria.* Available at: https://www.eatingdisorders.org.au/ (Accessed: January 15, 2023).

143 Lovering, N. (2021) *Orthorexia: 'healthy' eating can become an obsession, Psych Central.* Psych Central. Available at: https://psychcentral.com/eating-disorders/orthorexia (Accessed: January 15, 2023).

144 Crosby, J. (2022) *Orthorexia: When healthy eating becomes an unhealthy obsession, Thriveworks.* Available at: https://thriveworks.com/blog/orthorexia-healthy-eating-unhealthy-obsession/ (Accessed: January 15, 2023).

145 *Online treatment program for social anxiety* (2022) *THIS WAY UP.* Available at: https://thiswayup.org.au/programs/social-anxiety-program/ (Accessed: January 15, 2023).

146 *Post-traumatic stress disorder (PTSD) - information & resources* (2022) *Black Dog Institute.* Available at: https://www.blackdoginstitute.org.au/resources-support/post-traumatic-stress-disorder/ (Accessed: January 15, 2023).

147 *Online programs for stress, anxiety, and Depression* (2022) *THIS WAY UP.* Available at: https://thiswayup.org.au/programs (Accessed: January 15, 2023).

148 *Post-traumatic stress disorder (PTSD) - information & resources* (2022) *Black Dog Institute.* Available at: https://www.blackdoginstitute.org.au/resources-support/post-traumatic-stress-disorder/ (Accessed: January 15, 2023).

149 *Obsessive compulsive disorder (OCD)* (no date) *Beyond Blue*. Available at: https://www.beyondblue.org.au/the-facts/anxiety/types-of-anxiety/ocd (Accessed: January 15, 2023).

150 *How to spot 5 early signs of schizophrenia* (no date) *Psychology Today*. Sussex Publishers. Available at: https://www.psychologytoday.com/us/blog/and-running/202211/spot-the-early-signs-schizophrenia (Accessed: January 15, 2023).

151 *What is psychosis & the effects on mental health: Headspace* (no date) *headspace National Youth Mental Health Foundation*. Available at: https://headspace.org.au/explore-topics/for-young-people/psychosis (Accessed: January 15, 2023).

152 Neuroscience News (2022) *Inflammation may amplify effect of genetic risk variants for schizophrenia*, *Neuroscience News*. Available at: https://neurosciencenews.com/inflammation-genetics-schizophrenia-21781/ (Accessed: January 15, 2023).

153 Laura Lindsey Lecturer (2023) *Antipsychotic withdrawal – an unrecognised and misdiagnosed problem*, *The Conversation*. Available at: https://theconversation.com/antipsychotic-withdrawal-an-unrecognised-and-misdiagnosed-problem-196989 (Accessed: January 15, 2023).

154 *How to spot 5 early signs of schizophrenia* (no date) *Psychology Today*. Sussex Publishers. Available at: https://www.psychologytoday.com/us/blog/and-running/202211/spot-the-early-signs-schizophrenia (Accessed: January 15, 2023).

155 Hedrih, V. (2022) *Psychologists provide evidence for a causal link between greater forgiveness and reduced paranoia*, *PsyPost*. Available at: https://www.psypost.org/2022/11/psychologists-provide-evidence-for-a-causal-link-between-greater-forgiveness-and-reduced-paranoia-64233 (Accessed: January 15, 2023).

156 Cuylenburg, H.van (2020) The resilience project finding *happiness through gratitude, empathy and mindfulness*. Random House Australia.

CHAPTER 11

157 *Helping youth in crisis* (2023) *Sir David Martin Foundation.* Available at: https://martinfoundation.org.au/ (Accessed: January 15, 2023).

158 *Identifying risk factors* (no date) *Identifying risk factors - Alcohol and Drug Foundation.* Available at: https://adf.org. au/reducing-risk/aod-mental-health/identifying-risk-factors/ (Accessed: January 15, 2023).

159 Alcohol con*sumption, 2020-21 financial year (no date) Australian Bureau of* Statistics. Available at: https://www.abs. gov.au/statistics/health/health-conditions-and-risks/alcohol-consumption/latest-release (Accessed: January 15, 2023).

160 Alcohol, Tobacco & Other Drugs in Australia - australian institute of ... (no date). Available at: https://www.aihw.gov.au/ reports/alcohol/alcohol-tobacco-other-drugs-australia/contents/ introduction (Accessed: January 15, 2023).

161 Path2Help *(no date) The Alcohol and Drug Foundation - Alcohol and Drug* Foundation. Available at: https://adf.org.au/ (Accessed: January 15, 2023).

162 s c h e m e = A G L S T E R M S . A g l s A g e n t ; corporateName=Department for Health and Wellbeing; address=11 Hindmarsh Square, A. (2022) *Sa health, Alcohol use statistics.* scheme=AGLSTERMS.AglsAgent; corporateName=Department for Health and Wellbeing; address=11 Hindmarsh Square, Adelaide, SA, 5000; contact=+61 8 8226 6000. Available at: http://www.sahealth.sa.gov. au/wps/wcm/connect/public+content/sa+health+Internet/ about+us/health+statistics/alcohol+and+drug+statistics/ alcohol+use+statistics (Accessed: January 15, 2023).

163 *Nicotine* (no date) *Nicotine - Alcohol and Drug Foundation.* Available at: https://adf.org.au/drug-facts/nicotine/ (Accessed: 30 July 2023).

164 Path2Help *(no date) The Alcohol and Drug Foundation - Alcohol and Drug Foundation. Available at: https://adf.org.au/*

(Accessed: January 15, 2023

165 Causes and *prevention (no date) Can*cer Council. Available at: https://www.cancer.org.au/cancer-information/causes-and-prevention (Accessed: January 15, 2023).

166 *Vaping (e-cigarettes)* (no date) *Vaping (e-cigarettes) - Alcohol and Drug Foundation*. Available at: https://adf.org.au/drug-facts/vaping-e-cigarettes/ (Accessed: January 15, 2023).

167 Wakefield, M. *et al.* (2023) *Current vaping and current smoking in the Australian population aged 14+ years: February 2018-March 2023*. rep. Department of Health and Aged Care, p. 23. (Accessed June 3rd, 2023)

168 Australian Government Department of Health and Aged Care (2022) *What are the effects of taking drugs?, Australian Government Department of Health and Aged Care*. Available at: https://www.health.gov.au/topics/drugs/about-drugs/what-are-the-effects-of-taking-drugs (Accessed: 30 July 2023).

169 *Welcome · Mind Medicine Australia* (no date) *Mind Medicine Australia RSS*. Available at: https://mindmedicineaustralia.org.au/ (Accessed: January 15, 2023).

170 (No date a) *Drug facts - alcohol and drug foundation*. Available at: https://adf.org.au/drug-facts/ (Accessed: 30 July 2023).

171 *Online programs & tools for your mental health* (2022) *THIS WAY UP*. Available at: http://www.thiswayup.org.au/ (Accessed: January 15, 2023).

172 *Fentanyl* (no date) *Fentanyl - Alcohol and Drug Foundation*. Available at: https://adf.org.au/drug-facts/fentanyl/ (Accessed: 30 July 2023).

173 (No date) *The Complete Men Foundation*. Available at: https://completemen.org.au/ (Accessed: January 15, 2023).

174 *Federal government urged to ban gambling advertising* (2023) *Federal government urged to ban gambling advertising - ABC News*. Available at: https://www.abc.net.au/news/2023-06-28/federal-government-urged-to-ban-gambling-advertising/102534610 (Accessed: 03 July 2023).

175 *Sexual addiction screening test (SAST)* (no date) *Psychology Tools*. Psychology Tools. Available at: https://psychology-tools.com/test/sast (Accessed: January 15, 2023).

CHAPTER 12

176 Hay, Louise L. (1984) You Can Heal Your Life. Specialist Publications: Australia.

177 Seligman, M. (2011) *Flourish*. Random House: Australia.

178 Hay, Louise L. (1984) You Can Heal Your Life. Specialist Publications: Australia

179 . McKay, M. & Fanning, P. (1991) *Prisoners of Belief.* New Harbinger: USA

CHAPTER 13

180 . Cornelius, H. & Faire, S. (2006) 2nd Ed. *Everyone Can Win: Responding to Conflict Constructively*. Simon & Schuster (Australia) Pty Ltd: Sydney

181 . Kidman, A. (1990) *Managing Love and Hate: A Self Help Manual*. Biochemical and General Services: St Leonards, Australia.

182 . Kidman, A. (1990) *Managing Love and Hate: A Self Help Manual*. Biochemical and General Services: St Leonards, Australia.

CHAPTER 14

183 Hutchison, D.E. (2022) A Practical Guide for Self Change. Self-Published. Available at www.amazon.com/books/author/dianahutchison

184 Cloud, H. (2017) *Boundaries: When to say yes, when to say no, to take control of your life, Amazon*. Zondervan. Available at: https://www.amazon.com/Boundaries-When-Take-Control-Your/dp/0310247454 (Accessed: January 16, 2023).

185 Hutchison, D.E. (2022) A Practical Guide for Self Change. Self-Published. Available at www.amazon.com/books/author/

186 Miller, Caroline A. (2017) Getting Grit: The evidence-based approach to cultivating passion, perseverance and purpose. Sounds True: USA

187 Seligman, M.E.P. (1990) *Learned Optimism*. Random House: Australia

188 Seligman, M.E.P. (1990) *Learned Optimism*. Random House: Australia

189 Siegel, Daniel (2010) Mindsight: The New Science of Personal Transformation. Bantam Books: USA

190 Siegel, Daniel (2010) Mindsight: The New Science of Personal Transformation. Bantam Books: USA

191 Seligman, M.E.P. (2011) *Flourish.* Random House: Australia

192 Seligman, M.E.P. (2011) *Flourish.* Random House: Australia

ABOUT THE AUTHOR

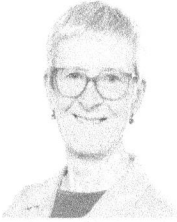

Diana Hutchison is an author, counsellor and coach whose life-long passion for self-development has led her to create a series of books in the self-help genre. Being drawn towards understanding multiple ways and modalities, she sought to create meaning for herself and her life which has meant that her unique holistic approach explores all levels of being: physical, mental, emotional and spiritual, leading to a perspective of self-healing which enables the best results for her clients. This multiple perspective has inspired the authorship of the Practical Guide series, of which this book is the second.

COMING SOON

Third book in this series:

A Practical Guide for Grief and Loss

To learn more about what Diana offers for your self-healing please visit www.dianahutchison.com and sign up for her newsletter. To be updated on her upcoming books, you may follow her on Amazon at www.Amazon.com/author/dianahutchison

www.dianahutchison.com/shop

www.ingramcontent.com/pod-product-compliance
Lightning Source LLC
Chambersburg PA
CBHW072040020426
42334CB00017B/1345